D0237516

Mentorship in Healthcare

Other books from M&K include:

**A Pre-Reader for the Foundation Degree
in Health and Social Care Practice**
ISBN: 9781905539680

Research Issues in Health and Social Care
ISBN: 9781905539680

Valuing People with a Learning Disability
ISBN: 9781905539666

Timely Discharge from Hospital
ISBN: 9781905539550

Perinatal Mental Health
ISBN: 9781905539499

Ward Based Critical Care
ISBN: 9781905539031

Preoperative Assessment & Perioperative Management
ISBN: 9781905539024

The ECG Workbook
ISBN: 9781905539772

Mentorship in Healthcare

edited by
Mary E Shaw and John Fulton

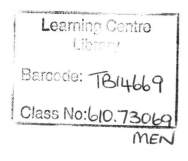
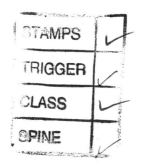
Mentorship in Healthcare
Mary E Shaw
John Fulton

ISBN: 9781905539-70-3

First published 2012

British Library Cataloguing in Publication Data
A catalogue record for this book is available from the British Library

Notice
Clinical practice and medical knowledge constantly evolve. Standard safety precautions must be followed, but, as knowledge is broadened by research, changes in practice, treatment and drug therapy may become necessary or appropriate. Readers must check the most current product information provided by the manufacturer of each drug to be administered and verify the dosages and correct administration, as well as contraindications. It is the responsibility of the practitioner, utilising the experience and knowledge of the patient, to determine dosages and the best treatment for each individual patient. Any brands mentioned in this book are as examples only and are not endorsed by the publisher. Neither the publisher nor the authors assume any liability for any injury and/or damage to persons or property arising from this publication.

To contact M&K Publishing write to:
M&K Update Ltd · The Old Bakery · St. John's Street
Keswick · Cumbria CA12 5AS
Tel: 01768 773030 · Fax: 01768 781099
publishing@mkupdate.co.uk
www.mkupdate.co.uk

Designed and typeset by Mary Blood
Printed in England by H&H Reeds, Penrith

Contents

About the Authors

Mary E Shaw MSC; BA; Cert Ed; FETC 730; RN; RNT; RM; OND.
Senior lecturer, University of Manchester, School of Nursing, Midwifery and Social Work

Since 1986 Mary has been in nurse education, including as a lecturer practitioner based in a large teaching hospital, and has taught on a range of health related programmes, including Mentorship, in face-to-face as well as e-learning mode.

Dr John Fulton Ed D, M Phil, M Sc, BA, RN,
Principal lecturer, University of Sunderland, Faculty of Applied Sciences

Since 1993 John has taught on a variety of health related programmes, including Mentorship, and has taken part in an international study developing a trans-European model of mentorship. He is interested in work-based learning and its promotion, and part of the core team on the University of Sunderland Professional Doctorate scheme.

Introduction

This book addresses issues around mentorship in the health professions. Whilst each professional group may address the issues slightly differently and even the same professional group's perspective can vary from country to country, there is a commonality of experience and of the skills and knowledge underpinning the mentorship process that transcends professional and geographical boundaries. It is at this professional and geographical interface that the book is situated. As such, it attempts to take a generic approach to mentorship and focus on the skills required for successful mentorship, whilst recognising the different professional requirements.

Mentorship is a concept that has been around since Ancient Greek times and clearly has a very long history. The term mentor comes from a character in Homer's *Odyssey* (Andrews and Wallis, 1999). The term has been used to describe the relationship of an experienced person with a younger more junior colleague; the relationship can either be a formal or informal arrangement between two people. The term and the concept have stood the test of time, and the meaning of an experienced or more senior colleague supporting and guiding a less experienced or junior colleague holds good across a variety of situations. In healthcare settings it is also used to describe specifically the supervision of a pre-registration student by a qualified practitioner with varying degrees of formality; for example, in UK nursing and midwifery the system is highly formalised. This book explores the mentorship relationship; whether it is an informal relationship or a highly formalised one, there is a commonality of skills that are required and the purpose of this book is to unpick these skills and the knowledge behind them.

As has been stated above, a different use of the term mentorship is employed in nursing and midwifery education, which has a very formalised system of mentorship. In clinical practice the student nurse or student midwife is allocated a qualified member of staff who is expected to monitor their skill development. The Nursing and Midwifery Council has become increasingly specific about the role and standards to which the mentor must adhere and in their 2006 document *Standards to support learning and assessment in practice* (SLAiP) they are very specific about the requirements for mentorship (NMC 2006). This also means, more often than not, a lack of choice in who the mentor is, which can present challenges for both mentor and student, as the mentor also has to assess the student and make an objective decision on progression. Of course, this is specific to United Kingdom nursing. Other schemes, and mentorship in other countries, will share the same principles if not the legislative approach.

Regardless of the degree of formality, mentorship is an important idea in health-care education, both in the initial period of training and in on-going professional development; it is important that the necessary support is given when learning through work in the clinical environment. To be fully effective, certain skills are required of the mentor. As an experienced health professional, the mentor will have the necessary skills and knowledge to practise as a professional. It is important that these skills are supplemented by the mentorship skills outlined in this book. It is recognised that the formality of the relationship may differ across different settings but the basic skills are the same.

Use of terminology can differ, with terms such as mentor, clinical supervisor and practice teacher at times being used interchangeably. Similarly, the term for the person being mentored may vary. For example, they are sometimes called learners, sometimes students, and sometimes mentees. Wherever possible the term mentor will be used to denote the senior colleague and the term student to denote the person being mentored.

Outline of the book

Chapter 1 explores the concept of mentorship and the ways in which it develops and enhances the professional development of both the mentor and the student. It aims to familiarise the reader, regardless of background, with the fundamentals of mentorship.

Chapter 2 examines the underpinning learning theories and teaching skills essential to the mentor's role and further examines how these theories can be used to enhance the mentorship process.

Chapter 3 explores the learning environment and examines the ways in which this environment can be conducive to learning, it also examines the notion of reflective practice and the ways in which this can enhance learning.

Chapter 4 examines essential mentorship skills such as communication, and the ways in which these skills can facilitate and enhance the mentorship relationship.

Chapter 5 examines the concept of assessment. Whilst those involved in mentorship may not all assess in a formal sense, many of the skills and knowledge outlined are generic to the mentorship role, as well as being of particular relevance to those who also act as assessors.

Chapter 6 examines some specific circumstances that the mentor may encounter, such as the student with special needs, the overseas student and the failing student.

1

Professional Development

Shelagh Keogh

The aims of this chapter are to familiarise the reader with:

- the case for engaging in professional development
- aspects of work-based learning
- the need for lifelong learning
- the sensitive or ethical issues which may arise.

Introduction

Since the early 1980s the term mentorship has been a word which is used with increasing frequency, and whilst there is a commonality in the usage of the term it does mean very different things to different professional groups. For example, it is used with socially excluded young people and refers to an older person who befriends them and assists with their integration in society, both in formal schemes and often in the more flexible sense of a young person assigned to an older person who will assist them in various aspects of their lives. As has been mentioned in the Introduction, within professional groups it can be used in a very specific manner, for instance, the role in nursing and midwifery education in the United Kingdom is one often more akin to a clinical supervisor who addresses a very specific and focused skill development. In other professional situations the term is perhaps used more loosely to describe a less prescribed and more informal relationship.

Whilst recognising the tensions in the use of the term mentorship, this chapter will focus on the notion of professionalism which underpins the concept of mentorship, and is common to all the health professions.

Activity

Activity 1

Reflect for a few moments on the concept of peer-to-peer mentorship.

If you have engaged in this activity, what were the benefits for you and your peer?

Consider also whether or not the process was easy or onerous. What made it so?

If you have no experience of the process, can you consider what benefits it could bring to your practice?

Mentorship as a principle

Whether used in a formal or an informal sense, mentorship is one of the key tools in use to aid knowledge management, skills development, and team building across the workplace. The practice exists in many forms, some formal and some informal. A mentor can be defined as a person who listens and gives advice to us for our professional development. More commonly mentorship is conceptualised as a top-down process but it also exists in peer-to-peer mentoring in formal and informal settings.

Our first encounter with advice of this sort is with our parents or guardians (informal), who teach us how to do what is necessary or is acceptable, in accordance with their understanding and their experiences, to develop our competencies and improve our knowledge. Moving on from this we encounter teaching staff (formal) that teach both in accordance with their understanding of their experiences but also in accordance with best practice documented in literature. The difference between the two encounters is that the first expects nothing in return whereas the second expects something; this could be in the form of tested progress activities or at least some interaction with the teaching. That said, even those who do this as an altruistic activity expect some feedback that their words are not wasted.

In the healthcare world during training, a lot of mentorship is experienced with the expectation of receiving judgements of progress and development at points during its execution. Generally the principle behind all mentorship is about giving or getting support for progress and or development during your professional career, both the training and the lifelong learning.

Peer-to-peer mentorship is a means of obtaining support which is usually developed from a trust environment in order to offer mutual development between parties. Some occupations or roles within organisations are such that individuals in certain positions can feel isolated and having an opportunity to discuss issues and ideas with someone who understands the common practice can be very liberating, resulting in a solution or an understanding exploration process. From this strand of mentorship **communities of practice** have developed.

A community of practice is part of personal and group knowledge management. The initiative provides a platform for workers to share, learn and discuss their understandings. There are levels of successful community of practice; rarely does this informal and formal organisation sustain good practice without some kind of management support. Some studies have tried to objectively measure efficiency and rates of engagement (Yang and Wei, 2010). A prerequisite to sharing knowledge is the willingness to learn. This fundamental requirement is easier said than done, take for example 'time management'. The majority of students have time management issues which cause great levels of stress, sometimes resulting in physical symptoms of illness, but do we learn from our mistakes? 'Rarely' would be the answer for most students and people generally.

Professional Development

As a principle, professional development is seen as a key feature of a truly professional person. Many professions such as nursing, law and teaching require the individual to demonstrate engagement with professional development as part of annual activity. Some of the professional bodies define mentorship as a feature within their requirements for continuous accreditation. As soon as one receives a requirement to do something, the shine of doing the activity may diminish slightly.

So why should we undertake professional development? One reason is that we spend a lot of time undertaking professional duties; therefore any contribution to the success of those activities will have direct impact on our lives, our job satisfaction and the lives of others. In order to achieve the best from ourselves, we will require a regime of reflection, by thinking things through, overcoming previous setbacks, capturing good practice and by benefiting from the experience of others. We are limited by the horizons of our experiences; as soon as we access others we can in principle double the knowledge captured. To access other people's knowledge requires us to communicate our ideas and thoughts with them.

One could argue that by reading this book you are committed to professional development but, if we ask a book a question it will come up with the same answer each time. If we ask ourselves a question we may come up with an answer which meets our desires rather than our professional need. Ask a respected friend or colleague a question and they are more likely to give you a different response based on their knowledge of best practice, hence knowledge is expanded. One can conceptualise a mentor as a respected friend.

Work-based Learning

Health professionals are expected to learn in clinical practice settings and engage in professional development activities. Whilst on some programmes a mentor is prescribed whilst others may choose to interact with a mentor, the mentorship relationship is a way to move forward without having to reinvent how to map the progression pathway. If the engagement with mentorship is focused around work activities then the term currently popular for this approach is work-based learning. **Work-based learning (WBL)** focuses on learning in and from the workplace where work, rather than a set curriculum, provides the focus for the learning programme (Durrant *et al.*, 2009).

Many organisations have incorporated WBL as part of their formal development opportunities. Some university courses bring together universities and work organisations to create new learning opportunities in workplaces (Boud and Solomon, 2001). Such programmes meet the needs of learners, contribute to the longer-term development of the organisation and are formally accredited as university courses. Work-based learning is seen as a means by which to support the personal and professional development of students who are already in work and the focus of the learning and development tends to be on the student's workplace activities (Brennan and Little, 2010).

Activity 2

List the people who have helped you in your development. Identify whether this was formal or informal.

For each of the persons above list the outcomes (learning) that you personally gained as a result of the mentorship experience.

Activity

If you have listed nothing above against the mentorship experience then one has to ask, were you an active participant or a passive passenger in the process? A prerequisite for gain in any circumstances has to be that the participants are willing to change as a result of the engagement. Even if you are in disagreement with advice given you have changed in that you have added to your personal body of knowledge in relationship to that particular piece of advice.

Reflecting on practice can be a challenging activity. Our understanding of our experience can be limited by our difficulty in accepting our weaknesses. Accepting our strengths can also be difficult for some people; this can be influenced through our cultural development. Hence having someone who can stand outside of the experience and return critical advice can be very beneficial, even if sometimes that advice is hard to accept.

Stakeholder involvement

Mentorship is not a one-way street in that the student is not the only one who gains. There are many stakeholders involved in such a relationship, the most obvious being the mentor and the student. In talking to individuals who have mentored others you quite often hear, 'I think I got more out of the relationship than the mentee'. Lots of knowledge development is in existence as a result of giving advice to others. In giving advice one has to reflect on one's own experiences. The reflection in itself is one interaction with the experience then the giving of the advice is a second pass on that experience, therefore it is not surprising that mentors gain a lot from the process.

Informal arrangements

It could be that students you have previously worked with request mentorship, so for example in my own practice people tend to look for those whom they have admired for the way they achieve outcomes and the type of achievements accrued. It has been usual to have encountered such an individual in striving for personal development, hence the commonality between the two parties. The potential mentor is usually very happy to provide this kind of support. How this works in practice depends on the efforts of the mentees to facilitate the arrangements. This type of mentorship falls under the label of informal arrangements; it could also be encompassed in the term coaching. In seeking out these types of mentorship arrangements one is also building up a network of advice givers to support future decision making processes.

Formal arrangements

With more formal arrangements, as in the case of UK nursing and midwifery education, mentors are usually allocated by management or by some formal process. This process is driven by procedures and requirements of the parties concerned. For example in nursing, mentorship is a prerequisite to obtaining fundamental qualifications.

The formal arrangements differ from the informal in that the agendas of each participant will be slightly different. In the informal arrangement the agenda is to explore opportunities for reflection and development only, whereas in the formal agenda there are many more stakeholders to consider, such as the following:

- student mentor
- mentor's manager
- clinical setting manager
- educational course tutor
- educational course management
- professional body
- Department of Education and Health (which pays for the training)
- the public who experience the results of the mentorship arrangements (more indirectly).

All the above would have an interest in the mentorship arrangements and would at some point want to know how the arrangements are impacting on practice and on the use of resources, be that time, people, places and money.

In order to be a formal mentor in an arrangement which covers professions which have compulsory membership of the professional body, an individual would have to satisfy the professional body that they have the competence to be in such a position. This is usually achieved by completion of an approved course as set out by the professional body.

Both the informal and formal arrangements have benefits as well as drawbacks. For example in the informal arrangements participants should consider conflicts of interest, limitations of participation in terms of time and areas of discussion, duration of interaction and many other issues. In the formal arrangements, whereby the mentor may have an assessment role, these informal issues become even more important.

Bray and Nettleton (2007) concluded that there was confusion in describing formal arrangements under the umbrella of mentorship. The following example will clarify this point, and the principles apply both to the formal and the informal aspects of mentorship.

Imagine you are a student radiographer and you are about to go into a clinical practice workplace where you will be given a mentor who will assess your competencies during and at the end of your placement practice.

Student radiographer – the student would see the mentor in a power relationship and as part of the management structure. The student's main objective would be to successfully pass the competency assessment and to achieve a good report.

Mentor/Mentor's Managers/Clinical Setting Managers – All these participants would see the student as a responsibility to look after but also as an aspect of professional duty, to ensure they meet fundamental requirements set out by professional bodies, institutional management and educational demands. The main objective would be to ensure that the student had a meaningful experience and conducted themselves in a manner expected of a professional person without taking up too much time or creating problems for other people.

Educational course tutor – this person would be responsible to the professional body, educational institution, and medical institution but also responsible for the student. The main objective would be to ensure the student was working in a safe environment which meets the student's educational needs. The tutor's role ensures the working experience does not reduce the effective relationship between the educational and medical institutions, produces the assessment documents required, and ensures that the participants have the right levels of training at the right times.

Educational course management – these people would have the same responsibilities as the course tutor but with the added responsibility to ensure sustainability of the practice and accountability of the processes.

Professional Body – this organisation would want to ensure that all students across their remit have equality of experience in clinical placements – very difficult to achieve when you have people involved.

Department of Health – the government would want to know if the money allocated was being spent in the right way to achieve the right results for the people of the country.

All of the above are accountable in law and have been taken into court cases involving practice evidence. Setting up a trust situation is very difficult if you know that at some point your words and actions could be the focus of the legal profession should something go wrong or someone else do something wrong.

The Public – who experience the results of the mentorship arrangements. The public's main criterion is the need to be in a safe place when they are ill and subsequently in a vulnerable position in terms of control of their own care.

Although the mentee has to contribute a lot of time and effort, the responsibility experienced by the mentor can be an added pressure and, of course, if assessment is involved the situation is further compounded.

Regardless of the formality of the relationship mentors are sometimes faced with students who are resisting change (we all can acknowledge that change can be difficult). The pressure to change can be misinterpreted by the student as a form of control. So the mentors have to develop skills to work with the student's approach to learning. To overcome the concept of power a mentor may develop a **horizontal learning platform** where both parties are learning from each other. They could adopt a coaching (encouraging) role looking for the mentee's strengths and building up confidence by increasing self esteem. The ancient Greek philosopher, Socrates, would mentor individuals by continually challenging their thinking so as to broaden the possibilities. Alternatively the student may work best in a very controlled atmosphere. The important aspect for the mentor is to get the best out of the student within a set time-frame.

Misinterpretations can also be experienced when dealing with different cultures. These cultures need not be so extreme as to be from foreign countries. Different regions, religions and sub-cultures in our own countries can have their own peculiarities and hence create different perceptions of the same situation. The spoken language in itself has a whole set of problems but body language presents yet another set of issues. One of the participants could be from a culture where too much eye contact is considered disrespectful; whereas the other participant may expect lots of eye contact in order to feel their words have been received correctly.

Lifelong learning

A further risk in formalising mentorship arrangements in the workplace is that it sets up a conceptualisation of how mentorship should be at the start of someone's career path. If participants' engagement is not just in the formal setting but also in the informal setting, they have a very useful resource to aid their development across their whole career lifespan.

To gain the benefits of any tool requires the development of skills. Professional skills required for mentorship are further explored in Chapter 4 Skills for Mentorship. As well as these transferable skills an individual can undertake personal development which allows them to gain from mentorship arrangements such as developing a personal standard or code of conduct.

During a student's programme of study the assessment strategy for their course will focus on certain areas that will drive a student's learning forward. If any individual wants to drive their learning through their lifespan then they should look for opportunities to assess themselves. Achieving lifelong learning depends on attitude, motivation and confidence (Cornford, 2000). The capacity of an individual to develop is within the individual; another way to construct this idea is to think about the term **locus of control**. The term was defined by Julian Rotter in 1966 as follows:

> **Locus of control** - *Individuals with a high internal locus of control believe that events result primarily from their own behavior and actions. Those with a low internal locus of control believe that powerful others, fate, or chance primarily determine events.*

We know that we cannot control life but we can contribute to our success by making the most of opportunities. At the end of seminars students are often asked what are they going to take from this class or what will they do differently or how will they think differently as a result of this opportunity to learn. Many of them are quite shocked that they are expected to think in this way. For example, after hearing about neurolinguistic programming many students find their ideas on thinking and learning have changed and conclude that everyone sees the world differently and that their views do not represent reality.

Recognising opportunities is a skill in itself. Lots of successful people have one thing in common, they are focused and always on the lookout for opportunities to achieve their goals. The people setting the goals may have set out a well structured pathway to achieve that goal. One thing is guaranteed, the pathway will have to change or at least deviate as it is impossible to control every element that will contribute to a plan. Therefore people have to become skilled at reflecting on plans against objectives and adjusting plans to realign to the focus necessary. Alternatively one may have to adjust the objectives; some objectives may have had to change due to the nature of the goal.

Having a goal is another tool which will drive personal development. For example you may have to undertake mentorship as part of your formal duties or training. You can tick off meetings on the list of things to do, chart each time you have a session with your mentor, or you can drive personal learning forward by setting goals yourself. Students usually find it difficult to set themselves goals but with a list of questions the process can be started.

Activity 3

Imagine you have been given the remit to set up your own job within your industrial setting, this can be your dream occupation. You might set yourself a list of questions as follows:

What would be the title of your job?

What qualifications would you need to achieve entry to this occupation?

From the list of qualification which one would you need to do first, second and so on?

How much would it cost to undertake these qualifications?

How much time would it take to be successful in these qualifications?

What would stop you achieving these qualifications?

Who do you know who currently undertakes this job or a similar one?

If the above questions do not help you, then develop a set of questions that does help you; remember active participation is the best way to learn. Lifelong learning is a common term used today; an important aspect of this is self-motivation. There are no specifics in this educational approach, each student would approach this in their own way; it is about personal character rather than technique (Cornford, 2000).

You will notice on the list of questions about your dream job that you were never asked about how much money you would be paid. There is a good reason for not including monetary gain in setting your goals. It has long been acknowledged that money is only the prime motivator when you are very limited in accessible funds (or at the lower end of the career ladder) but when you start to move up the economic security ladder it becomes much less of a motivator.

Discussions on Working Practice Issues and Mentorship

As healthcare professionals in the course of our working lives, regardless of professional group, we will be challenged in our beliefs and understanding, that is simply the nature of life. Especially in the healthcare professions each day personnel have to make decisions that test the boundaries of our comfort zones and understanding. Students generally should not be placed in these difficult situations but, if you have a student who is working with personnel who have to make these decisions then it is a useful learning opportunity to reflect on the situation. Building up the knowledge of others' experiences can help when in the future we are faced with similar situations.

An example of this from a mentor's point of view might be as follows:

You are working with some vulnerable elderly patients and one is particularly ill, not expected to last until the night. In the process of caring for this person the student considers the actions of professional staff to be less than caring. They feel that the staff should be with this person 24 hours a day and make sure she or he lives as long as possible.

You could discuss this with your student, exploring each stakeholder's actions against your view of the situation. Our views of the world as individuals are very different depending on many things such as, beliefs in what constitutes caring, attitudes to death and the right to have dignity and respect. There would be some core principles which are common across most practitioners but our interpretation of these principles sometimes changes our understanding in practice.

Ethical frameworks

A very useful tool to analyse a situation is an ethical framework. These frameworks are a series of questions for a user to ask of a situation in order to establish deeper understanding and a way forward, not necessarily the 'correct way forward' as there could be more than one way suggested by your analysis. Whether it is correct or not sometimes will only be established after application of a framework and receipt and understanding of the outcome; also sometimes solutions can be lawful but not ethical, alternatively solutions can be ethical but not lawful at that time. The most comfortable outcome is always ethical and lawful, bearing in mind the ethical struggle sometimes required to cross some cultural borders.

There are different types of frameworks, two examples are, **utilitarian** (aiming to achieve the greatest good)and **rights-based** (aiming to achieve the rights of the people involved). These tools will not give you the answer but will give you some good questions such as:

- Who are the direct stakeholders?
- Who are the indirect stakeholders?
- What are the facts?
- What are the laws relating to this case?
- What actions could be taken?
- Who would benefit from the different actions?
- Who would be harmed by the actions?

Your healthcare professional body will offer more information on frameworks.

Decision making in the healthcare profession does not have to be a life and death situation to make us feel uncomfortable, it could be simply a matter of financial constraint, time limitation or skills availability. Having a **case study** to focus on in a mentorship meeting can be very useful in order to give the meeting structure and focus and of course you can use case studies many different ways. The same case study can be used to examine ethics but very differently used to study developments of skills.

Throughout your discussions with students it is of course important to consider **confidentiality** so that you can build up trust between participants but there are occasions when this is not possible; if you think that someone is going to be harmed or an action is illegal in some way then your professional duty has to take precedence over confidentiality. Chapter 3 considers reflections and models of reflective practice which will further assist with the process of examining ethically sensitive situations.

Conclusion

This chapter has considered the concept of professional development and examined the ways in which mentorship and engagement in reflection on and in practice can assist with initial and ongoing professional development. This is an underlying principle that mentorship enhances the professional development both of the mentor and the student who is being mentored. In the following chapters these ideas will be developed further and the focus will be on the knowledge and skills that are required for development and how these skills can be used to support those whom you are mentoring.

2

Teaching and Learning

Mary E. Shaw

The aims of this chapter are to familiarise the reader with:

- theories of learning and learning styles and the application of these to mentoring in the practice setting.
- teaching small groups in an informal setting
- teaching a skill in a practice setting.

Activity 1

You may well ask yourself, why should you need to know about learning theories when what you do is teaching and assessing learners about your area of specialism? After all, in a busy practice setting, you probably show or demonstrate skills in the same way regardless of who it is that is being taught that skill.

If this is what you think, you are doing an injustice to the people that you train or supervise. Having some insight into these theories will enrich your teaching and instruction and enhance the students' experience.

Take a few moments to reflect on how you developed the skills that you are now proficient in. You will have had many different instructors over the period of your development. Did you learn all the skills in exactly the same way, or did the instructors take different approaches to skills training? Bear these experiences in mind whilst reading this text.

Introduction

The primary focus of this chapter is the adult learner. With few exceptions, you will primarily be dealing with adults aged from 18 years to those near to retirement. **Andragogy** is the term used to describe the process of adult learning, a term developed by Knowles (1984) who argued that pedagogical approaches to education and learning were based on researching animal and child behaviour and so were not appropriate for adults. An adult learner will have left school, and may have some work experience and also other life experiences and responsibilities, including those relating to family, domestic and financial matters. These will influence their approach to learning and how they learn.

The key here is that you will be teaching/instructing and assessing the performance of others, making judgements on how well they perform skills and demonstrate competence. Your assessment of that person will have impact on their future. The consequences for you are also wide ranging. Your goal should be to provide the learner with the best of experiences of instruction and assessment and to fulfil the function of a mentor.

Theories of Learning

Learning, be it new knowledge, a behaviour or a skill, results from a period of instruction that may be self directed or the result of formal or informal teaching or instruction. Learning is about some fundamental change occurring in an individual. Learning is a complex process and involves the senses such as sight, touch, hearing, smell, as well as an ability to remember, understand what has been seen, felt, heard or read. It generally includes being actively engaged in the learning activity.

Knowles (1984) suggested that adult learners are intrinsically motivated to learn, have a readiness to learn and have insight into their learning needs. Adult learners also bring with them a wealth of experiences that are there to be built on. These experiences include those of being educated and/or trained during their so-called formative years in mainstream education. Adult learners are self-directing and take responsibility for their own learning. The experiences they bring can be used to support group based activities such as discussions and problem solving exercises.

Learning by being actively engaged in the process has been shown to be effective not only in the classroom but also in clinical practice settings. It also enables students to link theory to practice (Wilkinson *et al.*, 1998). More recently Overton *et al.* (2009) found similar enthusiasm for small group evidenced based learning.

Learning theories may seem to be of little value to the busy practitioner. However, it is worthwhile considering something of the underpinning basis of how you do teach/impart knowledge in practice as it could help you manage the more challenging student. 'Challenging' may include the reluctant learner; the learner who seems only interested in technical skills and yet needs to be aware of the underpinning theory; the learner who is frustrated as they want to know everything at the beginning; the learner who cannot grasp what they have been shown; the learner who may have superior knowledge to you but has not yet grasped how to apply that knowledge. Look at Table 2.1 on page 00 for an overview of the four orientations to learning.

Activity

Activity 2:

Reflect for a few moments here about the most challenging learner that you have encountered recently. What made them challenging? Did it relate to how they preferred to learn or reacted to the instruction?

The Behaviourist School

Classical conditioning is perhaps the best known of the theories. Pavlov conducted experiments that resulted in an interesting response from dogs who were noted to begin to salivate when they could see food, before they began to eat. Pavlov introduced the sound of a bell with the food and later just rang the bell, no food being offered, and the dogs still salivated. The effect was noted to be transient unless accompanied by some reinforcement.

The teacher/instructor then needs to provide some stimulus for the learner that will trigger a desire for something, in this case to learn something new. There needs to be some reward system; this could be praise, a score for the task or allowing the learner to move on to a new level. Reinforcing the behaviour is important, though this is perhaps best when such rewards are intermittent. The rewards need not be positive, negative reward systems also work but this is less than ideal, for example the threat of some punishment for poor performance.

Table 2.1: Four Orientations to Learning *(after Merriam and Caffarella 1991: 138)*

Philosophies & Theorists	Major Concepts	Implications for Teaching/Learning	Ideas for Teaching/ Learning On-line
Behaviourism (based on Behavioural Psychology) • Skinner • Watson • Bandura	• Learning takes the form of facts, drills and practice. • Learning is evidenced by a change in behaviour. Behaviour is observable. • Responses are rewarded. • Modeling is based on observational learning.	• Teacher presents facts and skills. • Teacher-centered Teacher has 'The Answers.' S/he is the 'expert.' • Absolute answers exist in all areas of knowledge. • Students use mastery patterns in their approaches to learning.	Lecture notes are put on-line. • Text activities are on-line. • Teacher-directed. • Text is significant to support content. • Computer-assisted instruction (CAI) focuses on repetition, sequencing, and reinforcement.
Cognitivism (based on Gestalt psychology) • Dewey • Piaget • Bruner	• Learning focuses on the unobservable behaviour, the personal meaning making, generalisations, discovery learning, and coding. Choices we make determine who we are. • Truth and knowledge are conceived as personal and private. People 'know' things subjectively. • The nature of the whole determines the meaning of the parts.	• Teacher provides the structure for constructing individual knowledge. • Teacher and student share responsibility for active learning. • Audio and video tapes, graphic organisers, flow charts work better in this philosophy.	• Content is directed by the teacher from a variety of sources based in part on the needs of the learner. Web Quests are good examples. • Email • Computer-directed instruction (CDI) such as timed PowerPoint slides.
Humanism • Maslow • Rogers	• Acquisition of knowledge is followed by individual personalisation. • Metacognition (learning to learn) is taught. • Socialisation is important. • Values are in harmony with a spiritual whole.	• Teacher provides an abundance of resources from which the student can choose. • Interpersonal skills are highly developed. • Students become invested in their learning. • They try to understand another person's perspective as a way to learn the content.	• Teacher and students can both provide resources on-line. • Learning is tailored to content needs of the learner. • Audio and video conferencing are useful if technically supported. • Computer-aided conferencing works for the interpersonal side. • Discussions are central.

| Constructivism based on Gestalt psychology and cognitivism
• Vygotsky | • Knowledge is open to many interpretations and is in the context of a particular situation.

•Self discovery is a part of the learning.

• Students must make decisions based on their own values and sense of identity.

• Knowledge is the means to the end, not the end itself. It is based on a student's mental construct of a concept – that which they interpret themselves.

• Truth is relative | • Students use prior and current experiences to derive knowledge. Education is life itself, not merely a preparation for it.

• Teachers have to take the learners where they are and move them forward in an experience they value at the time.

• Students require more time to construct a concept than to be told it. Fewer topics may be taught but they retain it over time better.

• Hands-on activities work well here. Learn by doing is the axiom.

Teachers design activities and assignments framed in problem-solving. Role of facilitator. They provide support to start and gradually reduce support as student competence and ability to assume responsibility increase (scaffolding). | • Problem-based learning works well on-line.

• Use activities where synthesis of ideas leads to practical solutions relevant to student lives. |

The Cognitive School

This involves, according to McKenna (1995), '... internal purposive processes concerned with thinking, perception, organisation and insight.'

This suggests that the learner is engaged in thinking about the situation in hand and uses problem solving to bring about a change in attitude or behaviour. This process may be guided, nurtured and controlled by the teacher/practitioner.

Many cognitive theorists take what is referred to as a **constructionist approach** to learning. (See below in The Social and Situational School section, and Chapter 6.)

The Humanist School

As the name implies, this school of thinking is concerned with the individual and their feelings, needs and experiences. Maslow is perhaps one of the earliest proponents, with his work based upon a hierarchy of human need (Maslow, 1971). Maslow believed that motivation was key to learning and postulated that basic and other needs had to be met before the learner could progress to a higher level of learning, **self-actualisation**. The focus of educational activity should therefore be on guiding the learner through the phases of growth and development.

Rogers (1983), another humanist, was of the view that learning activity should be student focussed and experiential in nature. Much of the learning, he postulated, has to involve both cognitive and affective aspects of the whole person. The learning should be student driven, as is evaluation of that learning. It is these latter aspects that have brought criticism, especially where there is limited contact time available between the student and the mentor or where there are specific competencies to be achieved, and incrementally, as for example with a professional qualification.

The Social and Situational School

Bandura (1994) is one of the proponents of this school of thinking. The belief is that students learn through the processes of observation, imitation and by developing what he described as self-efficacy. Clearly then, this type of learning has relevance for the mentor–student relationship in that the mentor becomes a role model for the student to learn from in the real world of practice.

Lave and Wenger (1991) in their influential work emphasise the social aspects of learning. They draw examples from a variety of workplace situations and maintain that the learning process is a social affair and consists of learning or applying learning to the workplace and learning how to do things in the way of the '**community of practice**' to which the learner ascribes. It is an important part of the mentor's role to assist the student in becoming part of the community of practice and enables them to function within that particular community.

To some extent constructionist approaches are thought to combine both the cognitive and the social aspects of learning, this approach is further considered in Chapter 6. The basic principle of constructionist approaches is that individuals, rather than passively receiving knowledge, are active in their construction of this knowledge and it is the task of the mentor to facilitate the process; many of the skills outlined in this book are concerned with this process. For example in Chapter 3, the learning environment and the skills of reflective practice are considered.

Much time could be spent in arguing which is the most appropriate approach for mentorship; perhaps another way of looking at things is to consider the principles that would assist the mentor. Which ones are selected may vary from situation to situation. For example, in teaching a very practical skill the behaviourist principles may be appropriate. The humanistic principles may be more appropriate in setting up the learning environment.

Learning styles

Learning styles must not be confused with learning theories. A learning style is about the individual's preferred way of learning how to do something. This may vary depending on what is being learned. Many authors have written about learning styles and have developed tools to determine a student's preferred learning style and how these may be utilised to optimise the teaching/learning process. The problem with most is that they have not been scientifically tested and therefore their basis for use must be questioned. However, the underlying principle that people learn in different ways and take different approaches to learning is useful and is a good approach to take when exploring this area.

An example of this approach is the work of Honey and Mumford (1989) who suggest that there are four learning styles, namely: activists; reflectors; theorists and finally pragmatists.

Activists are 'get on and try it' learners. They will engage with the task in hand with enthusiasm and tend to engage in reflection on the task only after they have been through it. They enjoy a challenging experience but soon tire of it, wanting to move on to the next learning experience and may not have consolidated that learning. As a mentor or teacher you will need to consider how best to manage this type of learner. Reflect for a few moments about the challenges that this type of learner may bring. For example they may 'appear' more willing to learn something than for example the reflector. Share your thoughts on this with a colleague.

Reflectors tend to do just that, they reflect on or contemplate a task or experience, drawing in ideas from other people and resources as they do so. This may take more time than you have allocated and they might frustrate your attempts to get them to learn something in a hurry. They may not seem interested in certain aspects of learning, but this may be because they are still thinking about it.

Activity 3:

Again, consider a learner you may have taught that you can now look on as a 'reflective' learner. What were the challenges for you and how did you overcome these?

Theorists are sometimes considered to be perfectionists. They develop rationales and theories from what they observe in practice and have read about. They tend to be questioning about practice, and approach matters in a logical and systematic manner, preferring fact to speculation.

Finally, Honey and Mumford (2000) identify the **pragmatist** learning style. This type of learner is keen on theories; they are experimenters who like to put the theories they have learned about into practice.

Li *et al.* (2011) suggest that when looking at learning styles we also need to be thinking about the age of the learner when considering individual differences, for example, believing that the older learner is more independent than their younger counterparts but that the younger learner is more responsive to a mixture of styles. This view is endorsed by Vaughn *et al.* (2009), though it should be noted, they were studying female college students and therefore it may not be possible to generalise to the male population. In addition, many studies of learning style preferences have been conducted in western countries and may not be applicable to other cultures.

You therefore need to consider student characteristics when selecting your approach to their needs. See Table 2.2.

Table 2.2 Student Characteristics

Student characteristics (after Meehan-Andrews (2008):
Varying ages
Varying experiences
Varying cultures
Level of preparedness
Learning style

Activity 4:

Consider something that you have learned to do or learned about, in the past. It could be a skill you learned at school, in training for your occupation or it could be a piece of knowledge gained and used.

How did you learn the skill? Was it following a demonstration or instruction by a teacher/mentor? Was it something you read about or did you learn about it on-line? Was the topic easy or did you find it hard to master or understand? Was the teacher sensitive to your needs and did you like the teacher and the approach they took? At what age did you learn to do this?

You need to consider the age of your learners. At any age, a learner will bring some life experience with them and should be able to engage in the learning process. Depending on their experiences with practical instruction or any form of teaching, they will have developed some form of opinion about whether the experience was a positive or negative one and this could influence their approach to being taught by you.

It can be argued that the student is the person who has to do the learning. As teachers/mentors/coaches/instructors we only facilitate that learning process in practice.

Teaching a small group

Small group teaching is an efficient means of getting information across to several people as opposed to instructing each one in turn.

Having decided to teach a small group of learners on a particular subject it is considered essential that you do some forward planning for this. You could of course choose not do any planning but that could lead you to giving incomplete or incorrect information to the learners and in addition you may not think to include time at the end of the session to establish whether your teaching has been effective.

Overton *et al.* (2009) have established that small group teaching is an effective way to change practice and to ensure that there is an evidence base to that practice.

Planning for small group teaching:

- **Time: When will you teach?** How long will it take to cover the topic? You need to ensure you have enough time to cover the topic and for the session not to be rushed. Equally, do not make the session too long or the learners will switch off to the message you are delivering.

- **Where will the teaching take place?** A venue is essential and it should be large enough for the number of learners that you have. Make sure that you book the room and make note of where and when.

- **How many learners?** Is there a maximum number? You may be delivering a session to a handful of learners or a larger audience. It is a good idea to have this in mind when planning as it may affect how you deliver the session. For example, if you want the learners to undertake group work, this could be unrealistic in a lecture theatre setting. The size of the group may dictate how you choose to deliver the session.

- **What is the existing knowledge of the learners?** You should have some insight into their stage in training or experience in work. Without this knowledge you may pitch the session too high or too low for the audience. You also want to be able to build on existing knowledge. A way of establishing what the existing knowledge base is, is to do a pre-session test or quiz. This can be administered in advance or at the beginning of the session. You will need to build time into the session to do this.

- **Are you aware of any learners who have a specific learning disability?** It is a good idea to know about this to ensure the learner can access the venue or the materials you are presenting. For example, a wheelchair user will require an accessible venue and the dyslexic learner can benefit from getting the lecture materials a few days beforehand.

- **What is the topic?** Is it a topic that you are comfortable with or is it less familiar? It is worthwhile reviewing the topic and anticipating questions that may be asked by the learners.

- **What equipment is needed?** Standard delivery of materials in PowerPoint is the norm so you need to make sure that you have a computer or laptop and projector available. A laptop alone may be sufficient in a smaller room and with one or two learners. If you intend using a flip chart make sure you have somewhere to display the pages, this does not have to be a flip chart stand, it could be a display board or plain wall. If your session plan involves group activity remember to take the materials you need.

- **Planning to involve the learners.** This is a good idea in any session. Consider a variety of ways to do this: quizzes; question and answer; problem solving tasks. You will need to control how long they are given for a task and the amount of time should be realistic.

- **What are the aims of the session?** Plan to have one aim and several, not too many, objectives. This provides you with a framework for planning activity and gives direction for you and the learner and something that helps you to evaluate whether your session has resulted in student learning.

- **How will you establish that learning has taken place?** This can be tricky. Immediate recall can be good but then the learner may forget important aspects or they may fail to apply the learning. You need to decide whether to do a post-session test or quiz to test what has been learned. It will also show the learner what they have remembered and where the gaps in their knowledge are.

- **Evaluation of the session**, which may take several forms including: oral questioning; written questions/quizzes; observing the students using the information gained.

Teaching a skill/micro teaching

In the practice area you will be demonstrating skills or delivering a short lecture or seminar on a regular basis; you may well think that you do so in a constructive manner but how do you know that you do? Unless you plan for that teaching and seek feedback on your performance you can only 'guess' that what you have taught or demonstrated is effective in the sense that the learner has understood what the important issues are that you wanted them to remember and consider for practice.

In teaching a skill you will be demonstrating to the learner the ideal way of doing something and at the same time anticipating that the learner will remember the important messages that you wish to impart. The demonstration of the skill needs to be planned for. Exactly what is the skill? What are the component parts of that skill?; How much time will you have for the demonstration and how will you plan for the learner to practice the skill afterwards?

Preparation is essential: you need to know where you will be able to teach the skill with minimal interruption, for example some businesses close for staff training once per week, this might be something for you to consider. However, if there are several skills to be demonstrated each week, you need to make different plans so as not to disrupt production/activity.

The task needs to be broken down into its component parts so that you can ensure that the learner can see what the primary steps are leading towards completion of the whole task. You also need to be aware of the correct order (if there is one) of these steps, these should show logical progression in completing the task. Wherever possible, build on existing knowledge and skill (this may require you to find out about the learner's previous experiences by verbal questioning beforehand or the administration of a pre-session questionnaire).

You need to ensure that you have all of the equipment you need to perform that task, and if the learners are to practice after, this too needs to be taken into account. The cost of equipment may be a factor that you take into account when thinking about skills demonstrations. Because of cost considerations, there may be a temptation to use out of date items. Whilst you may think it obvious that you would not use expired goods in practice, the student may not and they may see it as the go ahead to do this in practice. This is sometimes referred to as a negative teaching/demonstration and is not considered to be ideal.

Do consider any health and safety (H&S) issues in advance, anticipating where your and learner's (and client/patient's where appropriate) H&S may be compromised, or where important H&S messages must be delivered as part of the demonstration. H&S considerations include not only the preparation and use of materials but also their safe disposal.

Ideally, you should practice the demonstration of the skill. This will enable you to establish whether or not you have broken down the skill logically; it will also enable you to work on your timing, not just for the whole but the parts or steps of that skill. You should also plan to establish what the learner has gained from the demonstration.

An important point is: do not expect all learners to be able to perform the skill effectively after this demonstration; for some, you may have to show them several times. You will have to think about what you consider to be a reasonable number of opportunities to see a demonstration and skills practice before you expect a competent performance. This will depend on many factors, including the complexity of the task and the number of opportunities to practice in the time the learner is with you.

You may wish to have a discussion about this with colleagues.

Activity

Activity 5:

Consider something that you demonstrate or explain to learners on a regular basis. It could be a skill or specific theoretical knowledge.

Exactly how do you teach/impart the knowledge?

Make a few notes for yourself about whether you have been successful or not.

Conclusion

This chapter has explored the concept of adult learning and how learning style can influence teaching in the 'classroom' or clinical/practice setting. Learning theories have been considered (though it is recommended that you read widely on this matter if you want to learn about the topic in more depth than here). Finally, small group teaching and micro teaching skills have been reviewed including evaluation of that learning but there is also additional information available on this topic in Chapter 5.

3

Promotion of an Effective Learning Environment

Mary E. Shaw and Kathryn King

The aims of this chapter are to familiarise the reader with:

- the characteristics of a good learning environment
- the ways in which the workplace can be maximised as a suitable learning environment
- approaches to promoting reflective practice in the workplace.

Introduction

In the previous chapters we have discussed some of the psychological approaches to learning and in this chapter we are going to develop the factors influencing learning by a focus on the learning environment and discuss the ways in which mentors can promote a positive learning environment. Many professional bodies require that a mentor or assessor should have specific professional qualifications, relevant to the area of practice. This registration should also be current. In such instances, holding an appropriate qualification is an important element of the assessment process as without it, the assessment is not considered valid. For example, in midwifery, a student midwife must be assessed by a Registered Midwife with the appropriate mentorship qualification too. Many programmes make it an essential requirement of the mentor that they have completed appropriate mentorship/assessor qualifications.

Activity 1:

As a practitioner/mentor/assessor, reflect on your own place of work and list both the positive and the negative characteristics of it.

Do you think that your place of work is a good place to learn? If so, what makes it so?

What do you consider students think about the learning environment in your place of work?

Make a few notes on these and other aspects of your place of work. You may decide that you will share your thoughts with a colleague in order to gauge their views.

Creation of a suitable learning environment

The creation of a suitable learning environment is a key to learners gaining an appropriate and positive experience when in practice (NMC, 2008). The Nursing and Midwifery Council (NMC) suggest that this involves the full utilisation of supportive staff and the availability of a variety of learning opportunities that match the learning needs of the student. It is easy to see how the same is true of most places where students are placed, regardless of the programme of study.

In UK nursing and midwifery programmes there is a highly organised structure which ensures standards are met in clinical practice and the professional bodies have introduced a system of audits which seeks to establish that the placement is a suitable learning environment and meets the learners' specific needs. In many instances, the education or training provider will have a specific template.

The following is an example of the types of areas covered by education audit in a healthcare setting:

- staff access to policies, procedure and guidelines
- availability of philosophy/mission statement
- the staff profile, including mentor availability (numbers and currently on the register of mentors)
- availability of a designated practice/education link person
- availability of health and safety information, including risk assessments

- reasonable adjustments for people with disability
- allocation of mentors to students before the period of practice
- availability of welcome pack
- availability and accessibility of education resources
- identified learning opportunities
- quality issues.

Whether a formalised system of audits is in place or not these are useful areas to consider when examining the quality of the learning environment. It is useful to remember that learning is a combination of the student, the mentor and external factors such as both the programme content and the external learning environment.

One of the main purposes of practice placements is to enable students to integrate the theory they have learned into actual practice and also to help them to begin to become socially integrated into the team. The learning environment is also about the resources available to support the learning experience. These include the people as well as materials to aid the learning experience.

Jokelainen *et al.* (2011) suggest that placement providers should prepare for the learner's arrival in order to ensure that the placement can meet the learning needs of the student. It is also an opportunity to identify who will be responsible for supporting the learner in practice, ensuring that it is not left to chance.

Student expectations of the learning environment

Students attending your workplace may or may not be employees. It is important to recognise this when preparing to support the learner. Evaluations by learners tend to highlight the physical aspects such as whether the place is too hot or too cold; whether or not resources are available; the busyness of the area. They also mention the atmosphere in the work place. They are sensitive to the welcome they receive and the attention shown to them when there. In his study, Lewin (2007) found that learners placed a great deal of emphasis on the importance of the 'atmosphere' of the workplace. Where staff were 'warm, friendly and relaxed and [there was a] supportive learning environment' this helped their clinical learning in a positive way. (Lewin, 2007: 244).

Learners tend to learn best when they believe they are made to feel part of the team and they are being supervised. This needs to be reinforced by the team being consistent and cohesive. Having a mentor who works with them regularly and who gives regular feedback on performance is considered best practice. The latter is not always recognised by the learner unless they are expressly told that they are being given feedback on their performance, so you should take positive action and plan for giving feedback.

It is worth considering at this point whether you will be supporting students who are not known to you at all or where the student is in fact your employee or work colleague seconded to complete a programme of study. It is possibly easier to manage the 'stranger' than someone you know.

Consider here some of the difficulties with managing a colleague for example. How are you going to manage the work boundaries and reconcile a different relationship that could involve the assessment of the performance of that individual that could determine if they are able to continue in employment? Chapter 5 deals with assessment matters.

Supporting Learners in the Clinical Environment

All learners have very different needs and it is part of the skills of mentorship to ensure that these needs are met and students should be given the opportunity to meet and discuss their particular needs with their mentor. An important aspect of meeting the students' needs is planning. Planning and preparation are key to learners having a good learning experience; this involves considering the various experiences which are available. The following questions are a useful framework on which to structure planning:

- Who are the learners that will be coming to work with you?
- How many learners will you have at any one time and for how long?
- What course of study are they on?
- What is their stage of training?
- How many mentors/assessors are available?
- What do they need to learn whilst they are with you?

This is a process sometimes known as **mapping learning opportunities** and matching them to student needs. All the staff in the practice area should be involved in preparations for the student experience. You should make use of team meetings to discuss matters relating to student issues. This will encourage colleagues to be aware that students are coming and when. It can also be used to identify support issues.

Carlisle *et al.* (2009) reported that mentors were benefiting from having students and preparing for their visits by developing training packages that they used to support practice. It is good practice to have a welcome pack available for the learner's first placement with you. These take several formats but generally they can include some or all of the following:

- A welcome letter (this could be posted to the learner or given to them on a pre-placement visit). This could set out the usual start and finish times; a contact number in case of sickness or late running; the name of the person in charge and the name of their mentor; a map or instructions on how to get to the placement; dress code.
- A placement philosophy or mission statement.
- An outline of the main activities in the workplace/description of what they can expect to see or be involved in.
- A list of resources available.
- A glossary of terms can be helpful, especially if there are some unusual words or phrases used in the workplace.
- Other relevant materials such as background reading.

Perhaps more importantly you must consider the needs of your patients or clients. They need to be aware that there are students in the workplace. If the students are wearing a name badge or uniform this may identify them as a student, but if there is not, then clients have the right to know that they are being seen by someone who has not yet achieved competence and in all cases, their consent should be sought to be seen by a student. Experience shows that few refuse to be seen by a learner.

Activity 2:

Take a few moments to identify the resources available in your place of work.

It is important that you think of the resources that will support these professionals but do not forget the most important recourse is the staff who can act as role models. Role modelling is not as straight forward as it might appear. Benner (1984) for example suggests that learners go through five phases in the development of expertise, based on the work of Hubert and Stuart Dreyfus.

Skill acquisition (Benner, 1984)

1) Novice

2) Advanced beginner

3) Competent

4) Proficient

5) Expert

Each phase of development is dependent on continuity of practice area, as well as a time continuum during which skills are gained. If there is a change in placement, for example moving to a new area, Benner (1984) suggests that the individual reverts to novice.

A novice is dependent on rules and applying those rules in practice, taking care not to miss any of the steps in that activity. They seek active feedback on performance. In contrast, the expert, it is suggested, does not follow all of the 'rules', safely cutting corners for a more streamlined performance. In addition, the expert acts intuitively. For example, if called by a student to help, they may delay responding and finish what they are doing and then attend to the call. On the other hand, an apparently similar call may be responded to straightaway as the expert senses that the request is more urgent.

This highlights that as an expert role model, you may not be seen by the student to be performing in the way you have advised that they should be performing. This can result in the student feeling confused about what is expected of them in practice. Try to be clear when instructing or guiding the student, about the standard of performance that is required.

Many professional development and education providers insist on an ongoing and effective relationship between the education establishment and placement. This may be in the form of formal links named by the institution whose responsibility it is to bridge the communication gap. Some may have a role that involves advising the placement on student matters such as progress with learning outcomes, or issues in respect of conduct or attendance.

As well as the people, you should make available up-to-date resources to enhance the learning experience. You may have included some or all of the following: textbooks; journals; equipment; access to IT and the internet; notice boards; charts; diagrams; information leaflets; other areas of the practice setting that could be visited to enhance the learning experience. By spelling out the learning resources, you are showing the quality of what is available for students; you are also identifying what is lacking and so can begin to build on what is available.

It is worthwhile spending a few moments here considering the obstacles that may interfere with the mentor/assessor/learner experience. Indeed, it is possible that you have already begun to think that some of the things suggested are not achievable. Why might that be? Reflect for a few moments on this and list some of those potential barriers.

You may have included:

- not having enough time to devote to the role because of work commitments
- pressures from management to achieve targets
- management appearing not to recognise the importance of, or the demands of, mentoring
- not fully understanding the course requirements or the assessment documentation
- previous evaluations having been negative despite the learner saying nothing to you on placement.

Your task will be to try to find ways around the barriers that you have identified.

Relationships in the workplace of the permanent staff have a direct influence on the atmosphere in the workplace and the efficiency with which people function. They influence how well or not learners integrate into the workplace.

Actually within, or accessible to, the learning environment there are likely to be numerous people who may be available to provide help and support to the mentor and the learner during placement. In many good assessment documents there will be contact details for people who can assist the mentor, for example, university staff such as module or course leaders and many areas have an identified member of academic staff who will assist the mentors in clinical practice.

In addition to these people, there may be others in the organisation who can step in to provide support, some of whom may have a designated educational role. For example, in the UK many of the large healthcare trusts have Practice Education Facilitators (PEF) and those studying for competence-based qualifications (National Vocational Qualifications and Scottish Vocational Qualifications) will have an Internal Verifier who will monitor the quality, usually at an institutional level.

Whilst each may have slightly different roles and responsibilities in supporting the placement learning, they are there to help and should be contacted as soon as a problem or difficulty is identified, or even if you think that there are going to be problems later on. You may have access to flowcharts that outline what actions you should follow when dealing with concerns. Look on your local intranet, there may be information there. If you do not have an intranet, you should be able to access the website of the education or training institution.

For example, in healthcare settings the PEF not only has a role in helping to develop the learning environment and giving advice on matters such as student capacity, they can also provide input on education matters, student and mentor support as well as development activities (Carlisle *et al.* 2009).

At some point in the student experience there will be some form of conflict arising from relationships with the learner. So called 'personality clash' is an example where the student or the member of staff just cannot get on with one another. These issues need to be managed in a timely way or else the student experience could be compromised and could result in failure to achieve learning outcomes. From a work perspective, it could also interfere with the business of the workplace.

Reflective Practice

It is important that students are given the opportunity to think about what is happening in practice and make sense of what often are unfamiliar experiences. Reflective practice can be defined as the way in which healthcare professionals learn from experience in order to understand and develop practice. Perhaps a way to define reflective practice for the mentor is to state that 'we all learn by our mistakes and by reflection can help others not to make those same mistakes'. Howatson-Jones (2010) suggests that reflective practice is based on experience and intuitive learning, learning that you may not be aware of at the time. However, bringing this learning into awareness by reflection is an important part of 'developing understanding, skill and competence as a practitioner at any stage'.

There are many reasons why we should reflect but here are some suggestions to consider and possibly add to:

- to identify learning needs
- to identify new opportunities for learning

- to identify ways in which we learn best
- to identify new courses of action
- to explore alternative ways of solving problems
- to escape routine practice
- to be aware of the consequences of our actions
- to demonstrate competence to others
- to demonstrate our achievement to ourselves and others
- to build theory from observation
- to help us make decisions and resolve uncertainty
- to empower or emancipate ourselves
- also for personal and professional development.

Across the whole range of healthcare practice, practitioners frequently face unique and often challenging situations and they therefore need flexible ways of responding to and learning from these situations. As early as 1984 Benner highlighted the usefulness of exploring critical practice as a way of linking theory to practice and reducing the knowledge gap. Today reflective practice is becoming more important, particularly as a significant component for the education of health professionals (Scanlan *et al.*, 2002). Dewing (1990) indicates that reflective practice encourages nurses to actively develop their clinical practice and expertise for the purpose of improving and enhancing patient care. In practice this means encouraging your student/learner to recognise that learning from past experience, whether good or bad, will allow their professional practice to advance their expertise. Reflective practice highlights the following sequence :

- things (experiences) that happen to a person
- the reflective processes that enable the person to learn from those experiences
- the action that results from new perspectives that are taken.

Although reflection is a fashionable concept, and in the past twenty years or so books have been written on the topic, it has a much longer history. Dewey (1933) suggested that reflection was 'turning a subject over in the mind', and Mead (1934) encapsulated reflection as 'the turning back of the experience of the individual upon himself'. It means thinking about what has happened and learning from that experience.

Ghaye and Lillyman (2000), for example, described the reflective process as being a transformative process that can change both the individual and the subsequent actions of that individual. Reflection therefore is a way of looking at your experiences with the intention of learning from them and with the possibility of altering your current or future practices.

It is easy to ask people to reflect on experiences but often a degree of structure is required to move people on from complaining to exploring the issues and identifying strategies to move on. One approach to structure is that of Kolb (1984) who developed what he called a 'cycle of experiential learning'.

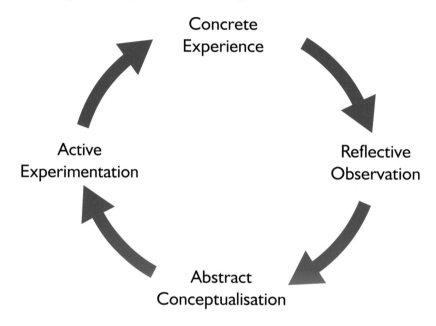

Figure 3.1 Kolb's 'Cycle of Experiential Learning' (1984)

Kolb's (1984) learning cycle shown above allows the student to reflect on the experience or the observation. For example the student recalls an incident or a situation; this is what is referred to as the concrete experience. This is followed by a period of thinking about the experience and relating it to the relevant theory; this is where the mentor may step in and assist the student with their reflection and in relating the relevant theory to practice. Fulton *et al.* (2007) suggested that people can start with theory or the abstract conceptualisation phase and then move into trying out ideas in the practical situation.

Schon (1987) suggested that there are two discernible types of reflection:

- reflection **in** action
- reflection **on** action.

Reflection **in** action concerns the way we think and theorise about what we are and have been doing as we actually do it. This occurs whilst practising and consequently influences the decisions made and the care given at the time. This reflective process may be entirely subconscious and automatic. Reflection **on** action is when we consciously explore our experiences in a direct and focused way. This is the retrospective analysis and subsequent interpretation of actions in order to understand the knowledge used and the accompanying feelings and frequently happens away from actual practice.

Another technique which can assist with reflective practice is the critical incident technique. Flanagan (1954) describes this as:

> Any observable human activity that is sufficiently complete in itself to permit inferences and predictions to be made about the person performing the act. To be critical, an incident must occur in a situation where the purpose or intent of the act seems fairly clear to an observer and where its consequences are sufficiently definite to leave little doubt concerning its effects. (Flanagan 1954: 327)

A simpler explanation is suggested by Mitchell and Everly:

> ...any event that produces unusually strong emotional, cognitive, or behavioural reactions in the person experiencing it. (Mitchell and Everly, 1993)

The technique of critical incident is one that mentors could usefully use with students, but it is important to bear in mind that students may find it difficult to discuss their experiences, especially when it concerns difficult and painful issues.

Activity 3:

Think of an incident in which you were involved in the past month or two.

Think about how you acted and answer the following questions:

1. Why did I do it?
2. Why did I do it in the way I did?
3. What other ways could I have done it?
4. How did I know I should do it in the way I did?

Activity

37

Having answered the above questions now ask yourself:

- What experience or previous learning have I drawn on to inform this experience?
- What new learning has occurred?
- What have I learned that I will be able to use in the future?

Perhaps better known is Gibbs's reflective cycle (Gibbs, 1988) which provides a very clear series of steps and questions which should be asked at each stage (see figure 3.2).

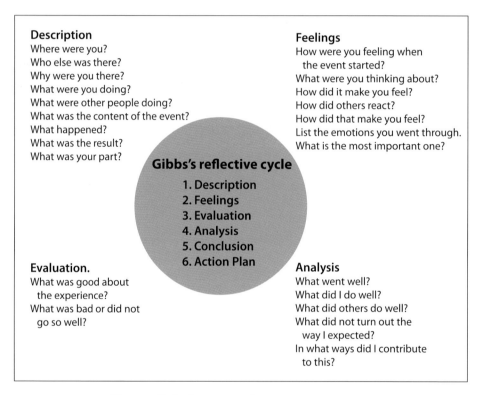

Description
Where were you?
Who else was there?
Why were you there?
What were you doing?
What were other people doing?
What was the content of the event?
What happened?
What was the result?
What was your part?

Feelings
How were you feeling when
 the event started?
What were you thinking about?
How did it make you feel?
How did others react?
How did that make you feel?
List the emotions you went through.
What is the most important one?

Gibbs's reflective cycle
1. Description
2. Feelings
3. Evaluation
4. Analysis
5. Conclusion
6. Action Plan

Evaluation.
What was good about
 the experience?
What was bad or did not
 go so well?

Analysis
What went well?
What did I do well?
What did others do well?
What did not turn out the
 way I expected?
In what ways did I contribute
 to this?

Figure 3.2 Gibbs's Reflective Cycle (1988)
(additional material adapted from Jasper, 2003).

All people are individuals and consequently the capacity to reflect is developed at different stages and in different ways in different people. The capacity to reflect requires time, energy, and motivation as well as commitment and open mindedness. The ability to reflect needs receptiveness to new ideas and to change and very importantly the ability to accept personal biases.

Enhancing Reflective Skills.

Atkins and Murphy (1993) discuss the skills required to engage in meaningful reflections.

Self awareness is about knowing yourself, being conscious of your own personality, beliefs and values, feelings, qualities, abilities and limitations; this can be difficult for many inexperienced people and the mentor can assist in this area.

Description of the incident is often the starting point and this requires a comprehensive account which captures the essence of the situation. This should include background factors, unfolding events, current thoughts and feelings and it is important that no judgements are made at this point.

The main idea is to move the person away from description to a **critical analysis** of the situation and the questions raised in Gibbs's model under analysis and evaluation are an excellent way of doing this.

Synthesis and **evaluation** help through the integration of theoretical issues and past experiences to move the person on and enable them to take a new perspective on the situation.

Activity 4:

Think about a recent situation in your professional practice, where the outcome was not what you expected, or where you felt uncomfortable about it.

Using the elements of good description, write about the situation paying particular attention to your feelings.

Can you identify a particular element that involved your feelings?

If not, consider the reasons why.

Talk through your feelings with someone you trust.

The reflective process allows the student to conceptualise knowledge and skill to develop self awareness. While there are benefits and limitations to each model of reflection, reflective practice has been identified as providing demonstrable overwhelming benefit to patient outcomes as well as contributing to developing practitioner knowledge and skill and informing clinical practice (Paget, 2001; Daroszeweski, 2004; Gustafsson and Fagerberg, 2004).

Conclusion

This chapter has considered several aspects of the learning environment: what constitutes a good learning environment, how to develop and also how to sustain an effective learning environment. It has also considered what reflection is as well as reviewing aspects of reflective practice. It has provided a structure and framework on which your reflections can be built and supported. It is important to remember that as well as reflecting on the mentor relationship yourself, these skills can be passed on to those who are being mentored.

The learning environment is not just the physical building; it includes learning resources such as the people who work there as well as the clients or users of the facility/business. Without these human and other resources, the learning environment would be sterile.

4

Skills for Mentorship

Catherine Hayes

The aims of this chapter are to familiarise the reader with:

- the skills required for effective mentorship
- approaches to giving feedback on performance
- the importance of documenting the mentorship process and outcome.

Introduction

This chapter will serve to address these key issues of organisation and communication by focusing on the best evidence to date of the experience of real mentor–student relationships and how these function effectively and rewardingly within healthcare.

The Individuality of Mentoring Contexts

It is the context specificity of the mentoring relationship which both individualises the experience and provides a raft of complexity in terms of how the process best operates. Within the healthcare and other practice arenas the distinct differences in approach to practice and how specific knowledge, skills and professional behaviours are developed are not easy to translate into a mutually defined relationship which encompasses all three elements of learning. However, there is a commonality of meaning and it is this shared and mutual understanding of what the process of mentorship is which will ultimately define the facilitation of learning and ultimately ensure the longevity of the professional relationship (Kostovich *et al.*, 2010) and will lead to a progressive and mutually satisfying relationship for both mentor and student (Jefferies and Skidmore 2010).

Specific aspects of the mentorship process include the following areas:

- how time is managed
- how challenging behaviour can be effectively managed without conflict
- how the development of strong interpersonal and communication skills can enhance the mentor/student relationship
- how effective mechanisms of feedback can be developed and realistically maintained
- how the documentation process can be governed and recorded appropriately within the guidelines of professional bodies such as the Nursing and Midwifery Council (NMC) or those professional bodies governed by the Health Professions Council (HPC).

Basically, this underpins the philosophy of mentorship which recognises the various social and professional transitions of both mentor and student (Kadivar 2010). By framing professional progression in the relationship, the role of the mentor should change accordingly so that at the beginning of the relationship the student is likely to be more dependent upon their mentor. This will necessitate regular meetings, regular feedback and a higher degree of commitment from both parties than at a later stage in the relationship when a high degree of professional autonomy has been achieved on behalf of the student. Ultimately this process will impact on the organisational elements of how the relationship will work and a mutual agreement of how best this should operate. In its most basic form it is possible to break the role of the mentor into that of an organiser and a communicator (Bulut *et al.*, 2010).

Activity 1:

With another person who has acted as a mentor within a discipline of healthcare, discuss the key elements of a healthy and productive mentoring relationship which you have experienced.

Reflect on key elements of why this relationship was successful in terms of:

a) positive and productive dialogue in the face-to-face mentoring sessions

Activity

b) parameters of the professional relationship

c) using your own expertise to inform a progressive development pathway for your student.

The Philosophy of the Mentoring Relationship

Whilst considering the individuality of mentoring contexts what is common and fundamental to every mentoring relationship is the philosophy of **social constructivism**, which is a driving force behind not only the mechanisms of teaching and learning adopted in skill acquisition but the motivation to achieve competency and proficiency in different domains of learning. A key theorist in this discipline was Lev Vygotsky, who advocated the notion that people learn through fundamental social experience and interaction (Vygotsky, 1978). This is particularly applicable to the context of mentorship where, essentially, learning and development are social and collaborative activities. As such teaching should be related to the practical situation and in terms of healthcare should be linked to patients and patient care as well as the experiences of the individual student.

Vygotsky (1978) refers to the *'Zone of Proximal Development'*, and by this he means the space between where the student is now and where he or she wishes to be (or where the mentor wants the student to get to). This is where learning takes place and where the student may need help or support. This is referred to as 'scaffolding' of the learning and this scaffolding is gradually withdrawn as the learner becomes more self sufficient.

The concepts of **connection** and **separation** are central to the development of the knowledge, understanding and value judgements underpinning clinical professional practice regardless of the academic discipline. The concept of connection and separation stem from the intrinsic motivations and agendas between the mentor and the student and this should be considered in terms of this relationship being mutually beneficial (Taylor, 1999). In essence:

- **Separate Behaviour** is the notion of objectivity and formalisation of ideas and the development of teaching and learning whereby the mentor will attempt to apply logic to the situation and be relatively closed to the exploration of issues beyond the parameters of the mentorship arrangement.

- **Connected Behaviour** is an approach which is empathic in approach which accepts subjectivity as a mechanism whereby the personal attributes of a student ultimately underpin their professional behaviour and that by aiming to listen and ask questions a greater understanding of the student's stance can be achieved.

- **Constructed Behaviour** is a holistic approach whereby the mentor is sensitive to both the concepts of separate and connected behaviour and can effectively utilise both approaches depending on the specific context of the interaction. In terms of the attributes of an effective mentor it is the constructed behaviour which gives a flexible and responsive approach which provides logic alongside understanding so that students are better able to socially construct meaning around their experience.

Skills for mentorship

Time Management

In terms of best managing time, synchronising a goal for achievement is the cornerstone of building a mentorship relationship (Clutterbuck and Megginson, 2009). One of the most important steps at the outset of the relationship is establishing what the student wants to achieve in relation to the work they are undertaking. For example if the goal is a piece of academic work, are they aiming simply just to pass or do they want to achieve an excellent result and in terms of either, how much of a sacrifice will they need to make in their personal time to ensure that this can realistically happen? In contrast, if the learning is about the gaining of practical competence, how feasible is access to learning opportunity and practice and how best can the mentor facilitate this process within the confines of a hectic clinical schedule? Other considerations like work-life balance will need to be discussed in order that targets set can be tailored and individualised for the student, so the whole process is not solely based on the task to be mastered but on the context and life within which it can be achieved (Anderson *et al.*, 2006). For example if a student wishes to maintain their social life then they might wish to consider which other aspects of their working life need to be compromised in order to ensure the focus of their learning can be achieved.

Charting time should become a mechanism by which students can map out mornings, afternoons and evenings and include weekends if they are not scheduled to work. Ideally all activities should be included and the more detail the better. Often an analysis of where time is being productively spent in relation to previously unidentified free time can reveal an opportunity to be focused on the learning process. For example if a student watches a popular soap opera four times a week then in reality sacrificing this will equate over the space of an academic year to around an additional 80 hours of potential learning time. Once established, these thirty-minute sessions will become a habitual and regular focus for the achievement of goals and targets. For some people getting out of bed half an hour earlier each morning might equate to a daily extra twenty minutes of study time per working week. Again, over the space of an academic year, this will equate to an additional 60 hours of learning time. The reality is that a commitment to learning will require sacrifice of personal time – how this is achieved ultimately has to be decided by the learner and cannot be either dictated by the mentor or used as a regular excuse by the student. Another significant aspect of goal setting in time management should be the allocation of contingency planning so that time is not so rigorously allocated that inevitable illness or emergency cannot be accommodated in the learning process (Thomas-Maclean *et al.*, 2010). Acknowledgement that devastating life events happen to us all and there may ultimately be the need for a temporary break in study should this happen may also be useful. Learning cannot happen as an abstraction to life – only as an integral part of it. Of course asking a student to time plan a year in advance on a micro level is futile, but on a fortnightly basis this is not an unrealistic expectation. However in terms of a broad overview of what they wish to achieve by certain stages of the academic year their academic goals should be clarified in order to assess their feasibility.

Negotiation of mutual meeting or communication times is an integral part of establishing a formal contract within the mentorship relationship. Some mentors and students may decide on an informal mechanism of communication such as regular e-mailing and supplementing this with meetings with a very formal and focused agenda. Depending on the learning taking place this might be reversed in the initial stages of the relationship with a relatively regular series of face-to-face meetings, which upon the development of autonomous skill may only need minimal communication in the later stages of the mentorship relationship (Allen *et al.*, 2009).

Most significantly, time allocated to the mentorship relationship must be decided at the offset and be broadly realistic for both parties if the relationship is to succeed. It should also be recognised that the mentor is not the only person who will contribute to the learning process, whether explicitly or as an implicit component of the process. Other practitioners, teaching staff, colleagues, work teams and family will all impact and provide support to the learning process and ultimately shape the professional role of the student (Bray and Nettleton, 2007). Whilst the one-to-one traditional approach to mentorship might be adopted, the contribution and value of other practitioners in non-formalised relationships should also be a valued and acknowledged part of the learning process.

Assertiveness Skills

One of the fundamental core skills of being assertive in a mentoring relationship is being able to maintain the core element of objectivity and this is true from the perspective of both mentor and student. As soon as the relationship moves into the realms of a subjective friendship then this is no longer possible, since the emotional bonds of being a 'friend' supersede those of being a 'critical friend' and this is where the traditional definition of a mentor as a critical friend can be misleading and misconstrued during the initial stages of the relationship. Setting the **professional parameters of the relationship** is therefore a pivotal stage of development planning in the mentorship process where an end point to the professional relationship should be established, regardless of whether beyond this formalised agreement the mentor and student stay in touch. It is also a mechanism by which neither party feels socially connected to the other beyond the context of the relationship. Whilst this may seem a detached and ambivalent approach, ultimately it protects both parties in the relationship and ensures that constructive criticism can be used as an objective tool for developmental learning and should raise no suspicion of personal criticism on behalf of the learner. It also means that the learner can take measured risk so that feedback can enable further development and educational growth within the confines of a framed relationship underpinned by trust and mutual respect on a purely professional level.

Being assertive does not involve any degree of aggression or power, it is used purely as a mechanism of raising issues of motivation, communication, challenging assertions and ultimately facilitating the achievement of goals. Through the experience which enables the person to undertake the role of mentor, it is expected that they can act influentially by providing a degree of candour and honesty, which might raise issues not previously considered by the student. This element of the relationship needs careful management since barriers such as potential professional jealousy on behalf of the mentor or a lack of professional respect for the mentor on behalf of the student can arise where a degree of professional distance is not maintained.

In instances where the mentoring relationship has become dysfunctional due to incompatibilities the skill of assertiveness can quickly dissolve subjective feelings and emotions, which can detract from the overall objectivity of the relationship. Such skills may also help to diffuse potential aspects of social interaction which may ultimately lead to the end of the mentorship agreement.

Depending on the context of the relationship within infrastructures and healthcare organisations, the relationship can also be a mechanism whereby the mentor can bring a sense of perspective to the learning process. This may be achieved by identifying and bridging gaps between what the organisation needs and what a student wants in terms of a personal and professional development pathway.

Interpersonal and Communication Skills

In an age of emerging technology, core skills of engagement within the mentorship process are fundamental to the development of effective dialogue which can inform and direct the processes of teaching and learning for students. Central to the implementation of this process are the facets of core interpersonal and communication skills.

The old adage that we have two ears and one mouth so we can use them in relative proportions is fundamental to the basic process of communication where an essential understanding of the person with whom you are communicating is central to the success of any dialogue. By filtering information and deciphering not only the cues of basic body language but also the thoughts and feelings of the student it is possible to more appropriately pitch dialogue to engage and motivate them more effectively. Essentially the underpinning philosophy of all active listening stems from the fact that communication is a two-way process and conveying information depends on a willingness to understand the other person in the relationship.

Listening effectively ensures that the other person is able to feel worthy and respected in the relationship. It is possible to sustain communication on a deeper level by ensuring that communication remains uninterrupted, and the suspension of value judgements on behalf of the mentor until after the conclusion of the dialogue means that eye contact can be maintained and the appearance of sustained interest in the student can be maintained. Ultimately a relaxed atmosphere for an open dialogue should be developed, which is subsequently easier to recreate in the next face-to-face contact. Also, when the mentor gives their undivided attention to the student, this actually encourages the student to sustain their communication as well as ensuring a very positive and open rapport. Fundamental to the whole process is body language and the physical appearance of being interested in the other person's conversation. The intonation of speech, tone and speed of the conversation are also significant factors.

A basic reminder of how the mentor should appear involves a clear demonstration of active listening skills by adopting various techniques, including:

Posture: by leaning slightly towards the student, the mentor can show a degree of attentiveness and also demonstrate a commitment to the dialogue.

Eye Contact: by maintaining eye contact this will demonstrate your interest in the student. Don't think about this too carefully though as nothing appears more disingenuous than moving beyond establishing eye contact into a prolonged and disturbing stare. Smiling can also be indicative of encouragement and sincerity and sustain the social element of the conversation.

Non-verbal Response: rather than engaging in extensive verbal responses, it can be beneficial to focus on slight nodding, eyebrow raising and gestures of acknowledgement, rather than a more direct response, these will all signal to the student that they should continue talking. It is also significant to remember that the less a mentor speaks, the more a student should feel at ease to speak.

Undivided Attention: by focusing solely on the information provided by the student, the mentor, in face-to-face contact should enable a seamless and continued logical flow of conversation and permit the establishment of a mutual dialogue concerning the issue under discussion.

Active Engagement: by being genuinely attentive and interested in people beyond the context of the mentorship setting levels of engagement are enhanced. Remember people are more attracted to those who are interested in them, and will pay more attention to what they are saying.

Self Awareness: self awareness is a key feature of positive communication and dialogue. Whilst keeping an accurate record of the process of mentorship is also a key requirement of the process, the mechanism by which this takes place will need to be carefully orchestrated to ensure that the whole relationship does not descend into a note taking exercise, limited by the poor dynamics of face-to-face contact. Being able to relax in a trusted person's company is the initial starting point for the development of any relationship and the mentorship relationship is no exception to this unspoken rule, despite the fact that unlike other relationships, the mentorship relationship might feasibly have a fixed duration.

Constructive Questioning: it is the concept of constructive questioning which has possibly defined the traditional role of a mentor as a 'critical friend'. Whilst general social conversation can be the driving force of any positive relationship, the parameters of communication within the mentorship relationship need to be closely monitored otherwise face-to-face meetings become both unproductive and unnecessary interruptions to the teaching and learning process. This also links closely with the philosophical origins of the process of mentorship which are heavily rooted in social constructivism.

Differentiating Personal Attitude and Professional Behaviour: acknowledgement that people can have differing viewpoints and opinions is fundamental to all relationships whether personal or professional. However this needs to be framed within the context of healthcare professionalism so that regardless of a mentor or student's personal attitude, there can be an expectation that during the relationship professional behaviour is to be a norm of both, regardless of prevailing personal circumstances. What can be useful in either instance is to incorporate the capacity for pastoral care as well as professional guidance into any mentorship relationship so that at times of concern the two can easily be separated and most appropriately addressed. There may be times where an aspect of personal well being ultimately impacts upon our professional ability to perform effectively but this is all an integral part of our ability to behave professionally at all times.

Another aspect in this consideration is in our ethically sensitive method of dealing with a diverse array of mentors and students who may be culturally, ethnically or religiously very different to us but who nevertheless should expect to be treated with respect at all times.

Constructive Criticism: assertiveness is a core skill in the process of constructive criticism but should never be used as a mechanism of conveying power in the mentorship relationship, which is a mutual relationship based on trust and respect. Balancing the ability to deconstruct a particular incident or experience and then reconstruct it into a meaningful learning curve can be hard for both the mentor and student and if not handled sensitively has the prospect of derailing an essentially on track relationship.

Most significantly the traditional role of the mentor as a 'critical friend' has parameters set at the boundaries of a professional relationship which may or may not lead to personal friendship beyond the context of a professional working relationship. Non-assertive students can often be regarded as passive recipients in a process rather than engaging individuals with the motivation to succeed within the parameters of teaching and learning. Similarly an aggressive mentor may quash the motivation of the individual and their willingness and ability to learn freely.

Enthusiasm for the Subject Area: being a mentor necessitates a degree of enthusiasm for the subject area within which the mentoring relationship is to take place and this can easily be evidenced with the professional profile of the mentor and the individual contribution they have made to their professional body, clinical discipline or workplace. These levels may also be indicative of the professional status of the individual but more significantly may indicate the area of practice that is a particular passion for them. In this respect a mentor may also be able to open avenues of professional contemplation for students which otherwise would remain undiscovered, perhaps as a direct consequence of stimulating and motivating the student to learn more about a particular aspect of practice. Nowhere is this more apparent than in the dynamics of face-to-face contact and it may well be that different mechanisms of communication such as e-mail or telephone become the means by which the most regular mechanism of communication is established where often it can be difficult to convey subjective feelings effectively but which will ultimately drive forward the intrinsic motivation (Chambers, 2010).

Critical Reflexivity: The concepts of reflection and reflexivity have become means by which it appears we can quantify all aspects and processes of being a mentor, but what is fundamentally lacking in this approach is the need for reflexivity to become a mechanism for initiating change in future mentoring relationships. The process of reflection is often limited to critical incidents in the mentorship, which is a missed opportunity both in terms of personal and professional development. The need to carefully consider relationships, communication skills and mechanisms of making future mentoring relationships ultimately more rewarding is one which is little addressed and under utilised in terms of acknowledging the progress made along the journey of being a mentor. Critical reflexivity may also be contextually linked to feedback mechanisms which have been adopted in the relationship. It is at this level again that personal subjectivity and professional objectivity should ideally be separated so that progression can be made in the mentoring process.

Giving and Receiving Feedback

Within the context of mentorship, giving and receiving feedback should become a mechanism by which specific feedback techniques can be used to develop better relationships (Lave and Wenger, 1991).

The whole concept of the term 'feedback' conjures up a negative connotation of being a euphemism for being able to personally criticise someone in their chosen area of practice. Contrary to this, within the context of the mentoring relationship, feedback should be a tool used to actively encourage both personal intrinsic motivation and core skills of professional development. By this stage of a student's career the formalised systems of appraisal and professional development pathway planning will probably be an integral part of their role within the context of healthcare.

Maslow was the first to emphasise the concept of motivation and explicitly link this to productivity and psychological well-being in the workplace (Maslow, 1971). Acknowledgement and recognition of a job well done is a fundamental motivator for future development and progression beyond purely giving praise. Each individual will have a preferred mechanism for receiving praise and it may be that whereas some students prefer their motivation to continue working hard to come from the basic identification of where they have best achieved and an acknowledgement of it, others may prefer a more explicitly constructed explanation of how they can perform to an even higher level next time.

Maximising the opportunity for a student to reach their full potential is the fundamental role of every mentor, regardless of the context of the mentoring relationship. The acknowledgement that within an organisational hierarchy all employees have room to improve is essential philosophy for a culture whereby everyone can feel free to build on the pre-existing achievement and develop further within a safe environment. It is this ethos which underpins the concept of 'effective professional development' (Nash and Scammell, 2010).

An alternative need for professional development can be to address an identified need for a student to significantly improve a core proficiency of their professional role or identity (Marshall and Gordon, 2010). **Underperforming** can potentially be another key way of describing this and indeed this is where the language of 'negative feedback' can begin. What is significant here is the acknowledgement that when it is necessary to mentor someone by providing this degree of feedback, it can become a hugely positive contribution to a student's personal and professional development when it is carried out in a non-confrontational fashion. What can be particularly effective is the identification of a weakness by the student themselves or within the context of their peer group, which they can subsequently use as a focus for improvement without feeling pre-judged in the whole situation.

Essentially feedback should be a two-way mechanism of communicating about someone's performance, which allows a significant mechanism of self reflection for the student. Often the temptation for the mentor will be to move straight into their general observations about the student's progress in specific areas (Clark, 2006). Whilst this can be wholly appropriate, what can often be more beneficial in terms of internalising the need to address a key area is by giving the student the opportunity to reflect on their progress by simply asking them directly which aspects of their teaching and learning they think they are performing best and having an open discussion about this. Even more productive is the opportunity for a degree of critical reflexivity where students can engage more fully with how they can fundamentally improve their performance in key areas.

Differences in personality are a huge consideration for the mentor at this stage as some students will find it difficult to accept praise whereas others will not be open to constructive criticism as readily as others (Barnett, 2011). Reflection can also be an invaluable tool when the mentor is not always available to give immediate feedback and for particularly emotive aspects of the teaching and learning process when a period of consolidated reflection can be useful. One aspect of reflection is the tendency of more introspective students to turn every issue into a potential critical incident and the tendency of more extrovert students to trivialise potentially complex areas for reflection.

Completing Documentation

The governance and regulation of the mentorship relationship is fundamental to the whole process and each professional regulatory body within the health sciences may have its own specific requirements for formal mentorship. In instances where there is no formalised process of mentorship, then minimally, dual signed documentation should exist as described in Table 4.1.

Table 4.1: Documentation

Mentor	Student
Contractual organisation for the mentoring relationship	
Time-keeping and attendance	
Managing the session	Preparing for the session
Ensuring the quality of support	Establishing learning needs and objectives
Monitoring the effectiveness of the relationship	Applying learning from the session
Giving feedback	Receiving feedback
Monitoring ethical and professional issues	Self awareness in pastoral issues
Keeping additional notes, as required	
Reflection and Evaluation on the Mentorship Process	

Notes should be succinct, legible and a copy of each set of documentation should be retained by both the mentor and student, with due regard for confidentiality in the process (NMC, 2010).

Developing Resources

Activity

Activity 2:

Imagine you have been allocated a mentoring relationship with a new member of the team that you have worked in for the last five years. Assume that this person is at the same level in the organisational hierarchy as you and is marginally more highly qualified than you but much less experienced. Discuss the resources you think you would need to fulfil this role.

There are so many excellent publicly available resources on the process of mentorship, for adoption in formalised mentoring relationships that there is little need for the essential reinvention of tool kits and resources for implementation (Macafee, 2010).

However what is absolutely imperative is that any process adopted is adhered to once the contractual agreement between the mentor and the student has been established. Another key aspect in the development of resources is the consideration of the online resources so readily available, which potential mentors might access in preparation for establishing a mentorship relationship. In this instance what is most significant is that mentors consider the potential validity and reliability of information in the public domain and engage critically with any published material before its implementation. The implementation of principles of practice, which at first may seem practically very useful, may have serious implications for professionalism if their evidence base is not rigorously established or peer reviewed in terms of appropriateness for application to practice, regardless of the healthcare discipline (Bhatti and Viney, 2010). It is advisable that whichever fundamental methodology within the context of the mentoring relationship is adopted, a copy of this is readily available not only to those engaging in the partnership but also to those moderating the process and the overall discourse and outcome of the relationship.

In terms of resources the 'human capital' which supports and sustains the mentorship process from the perspectives of both mentor and student also needs to be considered as a fundamental aspect of the infrastructure necessary for the parameters of the relationship to function well (Jones, 2010). As well as the physical resources and context specificity required to ensure that the mentoring relationship can be conducted, emphasis should also be placed on how and where the respective mentor and student can receive direct support from others who also add a depth of richness and a mechanism of support to the embedded relationship of the two.

Conclusion

This chapter considered the practical skills associated with mentorship including those relating to the mentor–student relationship. Time management has been addressed as well as the interpersonal skills required of the mentor. The importance of accurate and timely feedback has also been considered.

5

Assessment

Gail Sanders

The aims of this chapter are to familiarise the reader with:

- the purpose of assessment and what should be assessed
- the key features of design for effective assessment
- the link between academic and practical issues in assessment.

Introduction

No other aspect of the educational process receives as much attention from learners as does assessment. Assessment preferences can determine choices that learners make (for example, choosing courses that are predominantly assessed via coursework rather than exams). Assessment determines how learners spend their time, shapes expectations, affects motivation, and ultimately determines whether a learner is judged to have been 'successful'. Assessment, unsurprisingly, is at the forefront of learner considerations. Yet if we consider assessment from the other side, that of the assessor, we may see a different picture. Educators can be inclined to design courses or programmes of study from what may be called an '**input perspective**'; that is, they will consider what information or knowledge they feel the learners need to know, and build their teaching around that. Then when the programme has been designed they will consider how best to measure how well the learners have taken in all of that information (Gosling and Moon, 2002). For example, an exam may be designed to include one question on each of the topics covered in the course, or a portfolio may require a section for each class attended. Decisions on the type of assessment employed may be influenced by time available, how many students are taking part in the programme, and even by such things as rooming. Assessment is often the last thing on the educator's mind when a course is designed.

The dangers of this approach are that in reality it assesses teaching, rather than true learning. In this chapter we will explore what is meant by this statement, look at some of the evidence that supports it, and consider alternative approaches that may be used by educators to make assessment more valuable to all stakeholders.

Activity

Activity 1:

Whenever we design anything it is best to start by thinking about what we want it to do, i.e. its purpose, and assessment is no different. The Higher Education Academy in the UK (2007) presents us with a list of possible purposes for assessment:

- Classify student achievement
- Provide statistics for external and internal agencies
- Indicate standards
- Provide performance indicators

- Correct errors
- Provide feedback to students
- Remedy deficiencies
- Estimate students' potential to progress

- Consolidate student learning
- Help students to apply abstract principles to practical contexts
- Motivate students
- Provide feedback to staff

Consider these twelve statements. Which of them do you think is:

a) A primary purpose of assessment?

b) A secondary purpose of assessment?

c) Not a purpose of assessment at all?

Ways of thinking about assessment

'Classify student achievement' is perhaps the easy one to recognise here – it is clearly a primary purpose of assessment, and indeed the one in which learners tend to be most interested. In fact, all four items in the first column are commonly recognised as being a primary purpose of assessment when this exercise is used with tutors in staff development sessions. Those items in the second column are also well recognised as being a purpose of assessment, though often these are classed as 'secondary'. The items in the third column tend to produce most controversy and debate, and some will argue that some of these are not the job of assessment at all. However, whether we like it or not, evidence shows that from the learners' point of view, assessment always defines the actual curriculum, and they learn what they think they will be tested on (Biggs, 2003). It is precisely because learners are so preoccupied with assessment that it can be used so effectively to direct their learning and provide them with motivation. However, that in itself can create problems with the assessment process, which we will explore later in this chapter.

Let us consider for now that all of the above statements express primary purposes of assessment. The variety of the statements gives us an indicator of just how complex good assessment can be. It has many, sometimes conflicting, purposes, and a range of different stakeholders. Broadly speaking though, the process can be divided into assessment of learning, and assessment for learning.

Assessment *of* learning implies a judgement made about a learner's level of achievement at the end of the learning process, and so has a *product* orientation. This is usually called '**summative assessment**', which results in a grade or mark that contributes to the overall summary of performance of the learner.

Assessment *for* learning is rather more complex and the interest here is in how the assessment can facilitate the *process* of acquiring knowledge (Sadler, 2009). Perhaps we can best understand the importance of **formative assessment** by considering a practical example of how we learn to be good at something. Take, for example, learning to drive a car. Few of us will comprehensively understand how a car functions, but by taking lessons, practising, making mistakes and listening to the advice of our instructor on how to correct those mistakes, eventually we feel ready to take our test. The driving test is the summative assessment of our driving competence; but all of those times that we have to reverse around a corner, get it wrong, and try again arepart of the formative assessment. So practice, trial and error are an essential part of the learning process; learners should be allowed the space to make mistakes and learn from them without fear of being 'penalised' by having a mark attributed to a practice assessment activity.

Formative assessment can (and should) be built into a programme of study in a range of ways, from the very informal, for example where a tutor may give verbal comment on an activity done in class, to the formal, for example where written feedback may be given on a mock exam or test. Allowing learners to make mistakes in a constructive and safe environment is an essential part of learning; formative assessment can make a considerable difference to the quality of learning (Torrance and Prior, 2002). However, one problem that is often encountered with formative assessment is the fact that learners often fail to recognise it as a valuable part of the learning process, and this can sometimes mean that they choose not to engage, focusing instead only on those activities for which they will be awarded a mark or grade. It is the role of the tutor to ensure that the learner appreciates the importance of the formative activities by making sure that they are clearly and explicitly aligned to the course learning outcomes, and by ensuring that learners have the appropriate skills to learn from the feedback that they get from formative assessment (Irons, 2008).

So, we can usefully think about assessment in two ways:

- **Assessment** *of* **learning**: Usually completed towards the end of a course as summative assessment. In this type of assessment the stakes are high (failure or a low grade may affect the learner's future progress).

- **Assessment** *for* **learning**: Assessment activities interspersed throughout a course to provide a formative judgement on a learner's progress. In formative assessment the stakes are low; it allows learners to experiment and take risks without the pressure of grading that contributes towards a final course award.

At this point it is important to consider the issue of assessment in the clinical setting. Formative assessment is, of course, just as valuable in a work-based learning setting as it is in the classroom. However, as a work-based assessor you have a particular responsibility to ensure that experimentation and risk-taking by learners does not expose others to danger. Giving learners the space to learn whilst maintaining professional safety and integrity will depend on careful assessment design, which we will consider later in this chapter.

What to assess?

This chapter commenced with a consideration of the input/output debate in assessment, and made the claim that only the 'output' model will really assess true learning. But what does this actually mean in practice?

An input model of assessment will tend to measure the accumulation of information that has been imparted by the teacher to the learner. In this model, we can talk about learning being 'taken in' or absorbed. Then, at the point of assessment, the learner is considered to be successful if he or she is able to reproduce it in a form reasonably close to that in which it was presented by the teacher (Moon, 2006). Yet this is a model of learning that has largely been rejected by scholars in a range of disciplines.

The constructivist view of learning suggests that learning is about something more than simple accumulation of facts, and that true learning involves meaning-making and development, and changing of conceptions of knowledge (ibid.). Essentially this means that the learner is not simply an 'empty vessel' that we fill up with knowledge. Learning is built upon what the learner already knows and understands, and this in itself depends upon such things as past experience, culture, and values systems. In this sense, true learning is unique to each individual learner. They will absorb new information and transform it over time, through processes of reflection and internalisation, into something meaningful to them based on the building blocks that are already there. True learning is therefore a function of the individual's personal identity.

Pertinent to the issue of work-based learning, with which we are most concerned in this book, are Wenger's ideas on 'social learning theory' (Wenger 2008). Wenger discusses the learning as a process of engagement in the practice of social communities and of constructing identities in relation to these communities. In practical terms this means that a learner in a given 'community of practice', for example nursing, or accountancy, will construct meanings from new knowledge based on the context of the language and dialogues of that community. So, extending Wenger's argument, learning is an issue of learning to 'become' an accepted member of their chosen professional community and take on a recognised professional identity.

If we think about these two different approaches in simple pictorial terms, an input approach to assessment does little to determine the meaning that an individual has made of the knowledge presented to them. I like to visualise it as knowledge that has 'ricocheted' off the brain with little transformation. What little meaningful learning does occur is simply a by-product of the process (see Figure 5.1).

The alternative output model of assessment takes account of the individual transformation process and attempts therefore to measure true learning (see Figure 5.2).

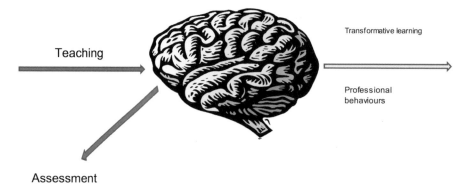

Figure 5.1 An 'Input' Approach to Assessment *(Sanders, 2010).*

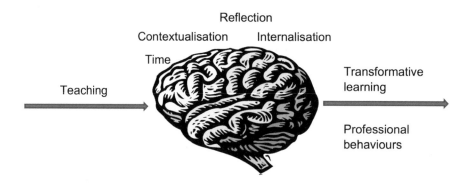

Figure 5.2 An 'Output' Approach to Assessment *(Sanders, 2010).*

These ideas are fundamental to your role as a work-based assessor, for they mean that you need to consider how your learners have made sense of the new knowledge presented to them, and how this has developed them within their community of professional practice. At this point, then, it is worth taking some time to consider what that means for you.

Activity 2:

Consider:

What do you need to know to be a good professional in your field? Write down the key areas of meaningful knowledge that you might look for in the people you are mentoring.

Activity

Meaningful knowledge comprises two key components. These are:

Explicit knowledge: This is knowledge that can be easily articulated; it will include discipline-specific knowledge and skills and is normally expressed in terms of learning outcomes, criteria, and level descriptors. It can be considered as '**knowing what**'.

Tacit Knowledge: This is knowledge that cannot be easily articulated and is learned through experience and practice. Take, for example, learning to ride a bicycle. Most five-year-old children can do this with some degree of competency, but they do not understand the physics that make it possible. Even adults cannot easily explain how they ride a bike, and yet they are still able to do it. In essence, 'we know more than we can tell' (Polanyi, 1998). This can be considered as '**knowing how**'.

Meaningful knowledge within the workplace always has these two components. Often the development and assessment of the explicit knowledge, for example, theory of pharmacology, accountancy theory, skills in using technical equipment, can be addressed in a classroom setting. This knowledge will be expressed in written *learning outcome statements*, and the way they are assessed will be expressed as written *assessment criteria*. Exactly how these are expressed will be determined by the *level of* the course. In the UK the Quality Assurance Agency (QAA) has developed 'Qualification Descriptors' as part of the Framework for Higher Education Qualifications (QAA, 2008). These are brief descriptors of the qualities of learning that will be evident in learners with named academic awards. You will find it useful to familiarise yourself with these descriptors before you design any assessment activities for your learners. Using these as the starting point, you may then construct learning outcomes and assessment criteria for any assessment where you are looking at the development of explicit knowledge.

Writing learning outcomes: Hints and tips

Learning outcomes are statements of what the learner can do or understand at the end of their learning experience. They should be:

- **Achievable** within the time available.
- **Unambiguous**: expressed in a language that is understood by all and is not liable to be misinterpreted.
- **Significant**: each learning outcome should represent a major achievement.
- **Assessable** by some reasonable and manageable form of assessment within the timeframe available.

(Adapted from Gosling and Moon, 2002)

Writing assessment criteria: Hints and tips

Assessment criteria are statements of how the learner's performance in achieving the learning outcome is judged. They should be capable of being measured or assessed in a valid and reliable way. A useful algorithm to use when writing criteria is:

1. Consider the learning outcome to be assessed.

2. Consider the assessment task set.

3. Brainstorm requirements for, or attributes of, successful performance of the assessment task.

4. If necessary specify the range to clarify contextual factors and level.

5. Focus on what is essential and categorise the requirements or attributes into clearly worded criteria.

6. Check that the criteria are measurable or assessable in valid and reliable ways and that the criteria are clear and unambiguous.

7. Repeat steps 3, 4, 5 until you are fully satisfied.

(Adapted from Gosling and Moon, 2002)

Learning outcomes and assessment criteria are designed to help our learners understand exactly what it is they need to do to be successful; however it is in the area of development and assessment of tacit knowledge that your role as a work-based mentor becomes really important, and this, by its very nature, is very difficult to express in written form. We therefore need to consider alternative ways of explaining to learners what they need to achieve to support the written statements.

Assessment for learning in healthcare practice

We all know of someone who has really good academic or professional qualifications, and yet is not very good at their job. Let us consider for a moment why this might be. Take, for example, a dentist. He or she may be very accomplished in terms of the skills and knowledge of dentistry itself, but if they are unable to comfort the small child who is terrified of the dentist's chair and cope with the anxious parent, or if they become stressed at having to deal with the financial accounts for the practice, or do not have the ability and insight to select the right people to work for them, then they are unlikely to be truly successful. Yet it is unlikely that many people who apply to study dentistry give thought to all of these diverse demands that make up the professional 'package' of dentistry. In any profession there are 'hidden extras' beyond the obvious skills and knowledge, and if, as assessors, we are to make a judgement about how effective an individual will be in a professional role then we need to include these both in our development of our learners and in our assessment. In effect, this means giving our learners the exposure to a realistic range of professional situations and demands, helping them to understand and develop appropriate professional behaviours within those situations, and then making a judgement on their performance.

We have discussed how meaningful knowledge comprises both explicit and tacit knowledge, and whilst explicit knowledge (and skills) can be taught, developed and assessed quite successfully in classroom situations, tacit knowledge development happens most effectively in the working domain.

Tacit knowledge in organisations has been widely researched and has been found to be a key factor in organisational performance. It is not uncommon for people who are highly successful in their occupations to have unremarkable academic records or, on the other hand, for those who were highly successful in school to be only moderately successful in their career (Wagner, 1987). 'Intelligence', as we normally interpret it, does not seem to be enough. An alternative form of intelligence has been postulated as a major contributor to professional success – practical intelligence, which may be defined as 'a person's ability to apply components of intelligence to everyday life' (Sternberg and Wagner, 1993, p. 518). This is the intelligence gained not through formal teaching in academic settings, but through informal processes in complex situations; the knowledge of experience; '**soft knowledge**' as opposed to '**hard knowledge**'.

Researchers have argued that the acquisition of tacit knowledge is fundamental to the development of practical intelligence (Sternberg and Horvath, 1999), although there is still a lot of argument about how tacit knowledge can be defined. Despite this, most researchers tend to agree that tacit knowledge is acquired through intensive personal experience and observation in the absence of direct instruction, and that its acquisition is highly correlated with success in the workplace (Insch *et al.*, 2008). Of course, sharing and transferring tacit knowledge is not going to be simple; we have seen that by its very nature it cannot easily be articulated. However, by considering how tacit knowledge develops and transfers it is possible to construct a model that we can use to expedite that process of our learners' acquisition of organisational 'know-how' and norms that help them to integrate more quickly. There are three processes of knowledge transfer that we are going to consider here (Nonaka 2007).

1. *Tacit to tacit*

2. *Tacit to explicit*

3. *Explicit to tacit*

1) Tacit to tacit. Development of tacit knowledge is a social process. Individuals acquire tacit knowledge from one another without the use of language (Baumard, 1999). It requires intense personal experience and happens most effectively when the learner is immersed in action using as many senses as possible (McNett *et al.,* 2004). Transfer occurs not through dialogue, but through action, observation and reflection. Ibarra (1999) describes the process of socialisation as the newcomer to the group learning 'display rules', such as appropriate mannerisms, attitudes, and social rituals.

2) Tacit to explicit. The conversion of tacit knowledge into explicit knowledge is effected through articulation. For example, discussion about the way a problem should be tackled will gradually tease out tacit knowledge to form a strategy or plan of action.

3) Explicit to tacit. The knowledge transfer loop is only complete when individuals can take newly-acquired explicit knowledge and internalise it in order to broaden, extend and reframe their own tacit knowledge (Nonaka, 2007). Only when the knowledge becomes internalised will that individual be able to access it without conscious thought and reference to codified explicit knowledge – it simply becomes part of the toolkit with which they are able to do their job. Internalisation can be encouraged through a process of reflection on action (Schön, 1983).

So, socialisation, articulation, and internalisation are the three essential elements in ensuring that the individuals that we mentor develop the tacit knowledge and behaviours to allow them to become effective members of our profession.

Socialisation might be achieved by engaging collaboratively with others. Since group norms and behaviours are best developed through a process of observation and experience, working collaboratively with a group will allow your trainees to observe how they do things and 'who is who' in the group.

Articulation can occur by talking through problems and issues. Often, even if we are unable to explain something in an explicit way we can gradually tease out an understanding by talking it over.

Internalisation occurs through a process of reflection. It is important that developing professionals internalise the things they learn so that they can use the knowledge almost instinctively. Essential professional knowledge must become part of their individual 'know-how' that provides the toolkit with which they operate on a day-to-day basis.

Using a model (see Figure 5.3 below) can help us to visualise these processes as a continuing process of learning that supports the acquisition and understanding of professional/organisational norms.

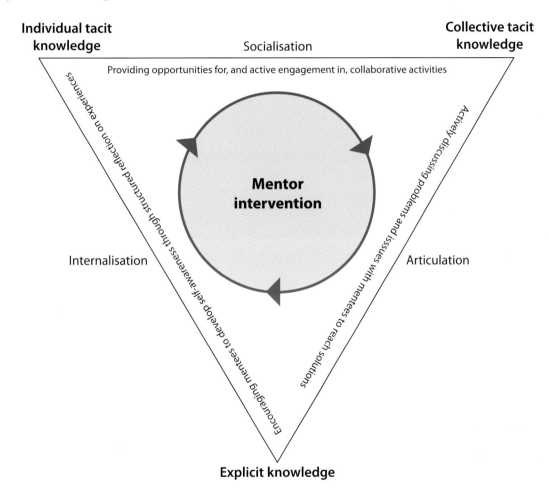

Figure 5.3: Learning Processes for Tacit Knowledge Acquisition
(Adapted from Sanders, 2010).

As a mentor you have a crucial role to play in making these processes work; firstly in terms of setting up the situations where learning can occur, and secondly in aiding the processes of reflection and internalisation by assessing workplace performance and providing feedback. Your interventions will ensure that your students will continue to move around the triangle, gradually growing their professional behaviours and competencies.

That, of course, finally brings us to the question of *how* to assess in a way that most encourages learning.

How to assess

We've already seen that most assessments are defined by a set of learning outcomes, and that these set out in written form what the learner is expected to achieve *by the end of a defined period of learning* (for example, a module, programme, or work placement). How the learners' performance is measured against these learning outcomes is normally expressed as written assessment criteria, which explain to the learners what they need to do to achieve certain grades or marks. This is all fairly straightforward when we are talking about explicit knowledge. For example, it is quite easy to assess if someone can work out a dosage calculation in a dispensary, or a sales forecast for a particular product, but what about the tacit knowledge and professional behaviours that we have been exploring in this section? By definition these are not easy to express in written form, either by the assessor who tries to write criteria, or by the assessed, who has to demonstrate how much he or she knows. You may have a head-start by having a set of professional competency statements which act as learning outcomes, but even these will contain subjective terms such as 'effectively deal with...', and it is your job to convey to the learner what this means and then to decide whether they have indeed 'effectively dealt with' whatever the situation demanded. Another question that arises from this is whether it is appropriate to try to 'measure' behaviour or professional competency. Is it really appropriate to grade someone as, for example, 50% or 75% competent?

Because of the largely tacit nature of workplace learning, often workplace assessment is a matter of *judgement* rather than *measurement*. In many scenarios it will be inappropriate to award a mark or grade (despite the fact that frequently you may be pressurised by learners to do so!), and your efforts will be better focused on using your professional judgement on how well the learner has performed. This then begs the question of how do you provide formative feedback on the learner's progress as they develop? For this I return to the development model above. Your learners will develop through example and reflection, and by engaging with them in a reflective discussion about their experiences you will facilitate their learning. This differs from the normal 'academic' approach in that, rather than control of the learning process being in your hands (as the 'teacher'), it relies on the learner being perceptive and self-critical, and being proactive in taking onboard feedback that you provide. In this model the learning process and the assessment become a *dialogue* between the learner and the mentor. So, it follows that you will be more effective as a mentor if you are able to *coach*, as well as teach in the more formal sense. Here, your formative assessment will take the form of a discussion between you and your student after each planned learning experience. By asking open questions you can encourage the learner to reflect on the experience and immediately correct any misinterpretations or misunderstandings that emerge from the dialogue. A useful format for this type of discussion might be:

- Tell me how you think it went today?
- How did you feel about what happened?
- What do you think went particularly well?
- Why?
- Is there anything you think could have been improved?
- Have you any suggestions that might help?
- What are you going to do now as a result of this experience?

It can be useful to ask your learners to produce an action plan from your discussion that you can review next time. This gives you a useful reference point against which you can assess progress.

The emphasis here is on moving away from the award of an artificial mark (students very often just focus on a mark without taking notice of feedback), to developing a system of assessment that will encourage in the learner an ability to self-assess and fosters a culture of continuous improvement. Inevitably, though, at some point you will be asked to make a summative judgement on your learner's performance, perhaps as part of a formal academic course or as part of a performance appraisal within the workplace. How and when you should do that is what we now move on to.

When to assess

The model that we have discussed above suggests that we should be assessing our learners' performance and giving feedback on an ongoing basis. However, this is not to suggest that we should be making *summative* judgements on their performance. The earlier discussion of learning outcomes explained that they were written as expressions of what learners could do or understand *at the end of* a specified period of learning or study. It follows that it makes little sense to carry out a summative (in essence, a 'final') assessment part of the way through this period. Despite this, the majority of Higher Education programmes are underpinned by 'continuous assessment' where students may be required to tackle a summative assessment sometimes only a few weeks into their programme of study. Some of these, in recognition that students are learning progressively, use so-called 'low-stakes' assessment early in the programme, i.e. the first few assignments may be worth a low percentage of the marks, say 10% or 20%. However, there is evidence to show that even using this approach, we are potentially disadvantaging some of our more effective learners. Sadler (2009) argues that the cumulative nature of continuous assessment often has the effect of penalising those students who learn more slowly than others, despite the fact that they may reach the same level of achievement by the end of the course or programme.

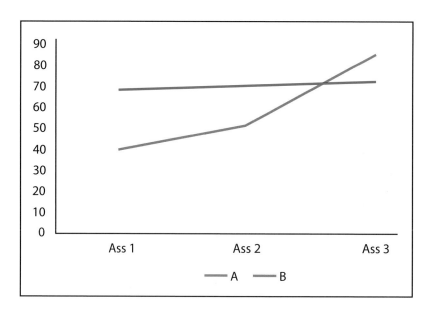

Figure 5.4 Learning Trajectories *(adapted from Sadler, 2009)*

He explains this in terms of 'learning trajectories'. For example, if we monitor the learning progress of two hypothetical students, A and B, we could find that A grasps the subject very much more quickly than B, but as the course progresses B's learning accelerates once 'the penny drops', and by the end of the course B is just as competent and more knowledgeable than A. Their learning trajectories could be expressed diagrammatically (see Figure 5.4).

Look what happens then to the final grade. Let's say that the assessor has tried to take account of the variability in rate of learning by weighting the assessments, with assessment 1 being worth 20% of the final grade, assessment 2 worth 30%, and assessment 3 worth 50%.

Grades	Assessment 1	Assessment 2	Assessment 3	Final weighted grade
Student A	68%	70%	72%	71%
Student B	40%	52%	85%	66%

A, being a faster learner, will achieve higher grades than B in the early assessments, and despite B catching up by the end of the course (which is really what we are interested in) he is not able to make up the deficit from the early assessment points. This may mean that two students, equally knowledgeable and competent, may have very different final grades, and this clearly does not reflect the true achievement of the learners. Effectively we are giving A credit for being a fast learner.

So, we have to be careful when we are designing our assessment regimen, that we are assessing true achievement and not some spurious performance measure that does not relate to our chosen learning outcomes. This leads us to the concept of assessment *fidelity*.

A note of caution: In healthcare, we may need to make sure that learners are competent to perform certain tasks for safety reasons before they are allowed to proceed to the next stage of learning. In these cases it is important to assess their competency at the appropriate point in the learning process.

Assessment fidelity

Ideally, all summative assessments that we make should reflect the learner's achievement of the learning outcomes and nothing else. Sadler refers to this as 'assessment fidelity', which he defines as 'the extent to which elements that contribute to a course grade are correctly identified as academic achievement' (Sadler, 2009.).

We have just seen that sometimes, simply through the design of the assessment regimen, other criteria that do not actually reflect achievement can creep into the process. However, often assessors actively build in these non-achievement elements into assessments, usually in order to control learner behaviour in some way. Sadler categorises these as 'transactional' and 'bestowed' credits.

Transactional credits are those that are included as incentives to encourage students to act in a certain way. For example, marks might be awarded for effort, attendance, or contribution to blogs.

Bestowed credits are those that awarded by assessors exercising their prerogative to grant marks for particular students because of some perceived special circumstance or disadvantage that the student has. For example, compensating for some acute health problem that the student has had during the assessment period, or making allowance for a student who is not working in their native language.

In most cases transactional and bestowed credits are awarded with the best of intentions, but nevertheless they mean that the final grade for that assessment will not reflect the achievement of the learner, and solely that. (As would be the case if marks were reduced for inappropriate behaviours.) Because the final grade or classification awarded to our learners can effectively determine how well they will progress through their careers it is incumbent upon us to ensure that it is a true reflection of their ability.

Activity 3:

Summarise the key issues which have been addressed in this chapter.

Conclusion

This chapter considered the purpose of assessment and has also explored the importance of assessment in determining whether the student has achieved the necessary competences and to the required level. Often, such assessment leads to a professional qualification or to determine the acquisition of skills for a role or job.

6

Challenging Situations

John Fulton

The aims of this chapter are to familiarise the reader with:

- aspects of diversity in the workplace
- the needs of overseas and home-based students
- challenging situations which can occur in mentorship.

Introduction

This chapter explores situations which the mentor may be required to consider, and like most situations in healthcare, whatever the professional background, there is rarely one solution which fits all (seemingly) similar situations. The chapter rather seeks to explore the areas of mentorship where extra knowledge or particular strategies may be required.

Equality and Diversity

Today's society is becoming increasingly diverse with people from all nationalities; alternative lifestyles are much more accepted than even ten or twenty years ago. Of course this is reflected both in the patient or client group and also in the healthcare or any other work force. However discrimination can exist, and be both direct and indirect. **Direct discrimination** means an individual in some way is disadvantaged because of some characteristic such as their race, gender or sexual orientation. **Indirect discrimination** is where the rules or working practice disadvantage a group of people; for example, expecting all male employees to be clean shaven can disadvantage people of the Sikh religion where the men are expected to have beards.

Discrimination on the basis of race, gender and disability is covered by specific legislation; for example, the current UK coalition government have passed an Equality Act (2010), which aims to consolidate the array of anti-discrimination legislation. This legislation aims to protect the rights of individuals against 'direct and indirect discrimination, harassment and victimisation in services and public functions; premises; work; education; associations, and transport'.

There are many diverse people and sets of circumstances in mentorship and no two will be alike. The key principle is, as stated about teaching, 'good teaching is good teaching' (Biggs, 1999), and the same can be applied to mentorship, 'good mentorship is good mentorship' regardless of the people and the set of circumstances. The situations which will be considered in this chapter are:

- the overseas student or the student whose first language is not English
- the student with special needs
- the failing student.

It is important that we celebrate diversity and draw from a wide range of people, it is also important that we are aware of possible ways of discrimination. We need to be actively aware of these issues for our patients or clients; it is also important that as mentors we are aware of the diverse needs of our students and potential students. This chapter aims to pick up on these issues and to explore situations which the mentor might find challenging.

Students from overseas

There is an increasing number of experienced health professionals coming from overseas countries into the UK, both to universities and the NHS. Others coming to this country wish to embark on professional training in one of the health professions. Many people coming from overseas are highly skilled and well qualified in their own discipline. The various professional bodies stipulate certain English language proficiency standards and a period of adaptation is required before the individual can obtain professional registration.

Students are individuals and overseas students are no different; they come from a diverse range of cultures, backgrounds and social classes. This means in practice that overseas students will have different expectations and needs. In particular, the background or demographic characteristics of the individual student, and especially personal characteristics, may be found to determine the way in which study is approached, and many experience difficulties in adapting to a western style of teaching and expectations (Luzio-Lockett 1998). Luzio-Lockett expresses this as the 'squeezing effect': the identity is squeezed as they have to express themselves in unfamiliar ways, which can have an effect on their performance. It can, therefore, be difficult for the student when they come to an unfamiliar country with unfamiliar working practices; people can experience a kind of 'culture shock' (Furnham & Bochner, 1986) which in its extreme form can lead to depression, anxiety and even physical illness. Most people do get over this and start to function independently, but the initial support that can be required should not be underestimated.

Also, the motivation and reasons for students undertaking study can and will significantly impact on their approach and ways of engagement. The majority of people come to this country to improve their skills and experience new ways of working. Many very skilled people come because of higher salaries and/or better working conditions. Others wish to support their families and higher salaries allow this. There is nothing wrong with any of these reasons and indeed many of our overseas colleagues have added much to our healthcare system and shown us how important it is to celebrate diversity.

Whether a qualified professional or someone commencing their professional training, students require generic skills, language skills, time management, the ability to retrieve information both formally and informally. All courses have language standards as entry requirements and students are expected to achieve this standard before coming on the course, but it is not quite as simple as it may first appear. Cammish (1997) explores the relationship between language and culture and argues that much English teaching (outside of Europe) may not be done in a culturally sensitive manner and whilst people may understand the words and their literal meaning, specific connotations may be difficult for the learner. In practice this might mean many of the concepts we understand and take for granted are often strange and unfamiliar to people from different nationalities. An example of this is the idea of snow, whilst people in warmer climates will know what snow is they will never have experienced or appreciate how unpleasant snow can be when it gets to the slushy stage!

This idea has implications when you consider that people learn new ideas in relation to those things which are familiar to them. Nasir and Hand (2006) take an overview of sociocultural perspectives and race, culture and learning. Not to oversimplify a complex and scholarly paper, they argue that people learn by relating the new knowledge to something familiar to them, often something culturally specific. In learning we often relate new ideas or concepts to a familiar experience, and it is important to get the student to do the same. It is therefore very important to remember that students may not share our experiences.

Another major issue is the approach to study; in academic programmes in the UK, the focus is very much on promoting **deep learning** as opposed to **surface learning** in students (Marton & Salvo, 1976a and b). The basic idea behind this is that things can be learned either in a superficial way or, in the case of deep learning, a way in which the underlying principles are fully understood or there is a change in the cognitive structures of the individual learner. Scardamalia *et al.* (1992) have described this as surface learning or 'knowledge telling' where the student can quote the relevant facts but may not fully understand them; and 'deep learning' is knowledge transforming when the knowledge becomes part of the way in which the student looks at the world. In practice based disciplines, approaches to learning can influence the ease with which knowledge can be translated into practice. Most students experience difficulties in engaging in deep learning and the overseas student is no different.

It is also important to remember that students from overseas may have had very different educational experiences from their British colleagues and the 'teacher' can be a very different concept; for example in the UK we encourage students to challenge and debate, whereas in other cultures the relationship is hierarchical (Galtung, 1981).

Cortazzi and Jin (1997) focus on Chinese culture and highlight a number of differences between British and Chinese approaches to education. In the UK the learners are expected to engage in critical debate, and demonstrate creativity and originality. The teachers are seen as equal to the learners. In Chinese education there is a hierarchical teacher–student relationship and the learner is expected to take a passive role and accepts what the teacher says rather than challenges.

In practice, this means students are used to different ways of learning and see their teachers in different ways. In the Western world the students often challenge the mentor and will state when they do not understand an idea or are unsure; in other cultures students are not prepared to question or challenge the teacher or mentor, and this is worth bearing in mind when talking to students.

Learning is a social activity and people learn in a 'community of practice' (Lave & Wenger, 1991). So the learning process is not just about learning knowledge and skills but it is also about learning how the particular area of practice functions, how things are done and what is acceptable and unacceptable. This process is part of being a student and can take time. As well as working with pre-registration students, mentors are often expected to mentor qualified practitioners from overseas doing an 'adaptation' programme. Whilst the overseas qualified practitioner will share an area of professional practice, approaches can and will vary from country to country. It is worth spending time and finding out about the different learning experiences of people, which can vary from country to country, and not making too many assumptions but rather gaining some understanding of the diversity of learning experiences.

Activity 1:

We have highlighted a number of difficulties which students may experience; what strategies do you think you can use to address these issues?

Expectations of mentors and students

It is worth bearing in mind that we need to treat all students as individuals and be clear about their expectations of us and ours of them.

- Expectations need to be made clear to the learner.
- Encourage students to take an overview of their learning and a sense of how they are learning.
- Use the principles of 'scaffolding' (see Chapter 4), provide support and gradually withdraw this support as students become more and more self sufficient (Biggs, 1999).

There is a body of work drawn from the experience of ethnic groups considering mainly school based education in the USA referred to as *culturally sensitive teaching* (Gay, 2000). It is mainly based on work with children and High School students. However many of these principles can be applied to the adult learner and they are often simple and easy to implement but can make a huge difference with the learners. It is important to remember (the obvious!) we are all cultural beings with our own set of expectations and beliefs; we are all very good at thinking that everyone should share these beliefs and views and of course people don't; it is often worth taking a few minutes to remember this. Following on from this it is important to bear in mind that people from different countries or cultures who do an overseas nurses programme may have very different educational experiences to our own. We should also try to draw on the experience of the students who will have done things differently in other countries; it is also a balance between not being too patronising and making too many assumptions.

The Failing Student

Whilst understanding of terms and how mentorship is implemented in practice varies from country to country, and professional group to professional group, one commonality is the difficulties and challenges of dealing with students who are failing to achieve. This type of student does present very particular needs and opportunities. It is very important to remember that not all who are having difficulties or who are underperforming are failing or are totally unsuitable for their particular chosen profession. Many will need help and encouragement and difficulties can be rectified.

The first principle is the importance of identifying weak students early on in their placement and getting the necessary support in place as early in the placement as is possible (Duffy, 2004). It is also very important to remember that most of the health professions, and other employment settings, consist of a diverse range of activities and it is likely that many students will struggle with one. For some it might be an aspect of technical proficiency, whilst for others it may be interpersonal skills. Regardless, the identification of weakness and the formulation of an action plan can do much to address these issues. It is very important to differentiate between people who might find an aspect of practice difficult or challenging and those who are unsuited for the profession in which they are studying.

Another issue is when someone does not agree with us or dress in the way we like, does this mean that they will not be a good professional? One mentor made this comment about a student:

How do you stand if, you know, I mean I have pulled students up for having a lot of earrings in or denims on or things like that? But sometimes I mean I have read different things where it's difficult to know if they have got bright orange hair sticking up in a Mohican or something. Is that their right to have that or are you within your rights to say 'that is not the impression I want my patients to have?'

(Source: personal communication)

Now this particular student may not have had difficulties with competencies but arguably his or her appearance was inappropriate and a different track needs to be taken; perhaps a discussion on professionalism and the impact lack of this can have on the patient's experience of care.

Activity

Activity 2:

Again, we have highlighted a number of difficulties which students may experience; what strategies do you think you can use to address these issues?

Shakespeare and Webb (2008) provide an interesting and thought provoking paper on mentorship based on a small scale research study. They discuss the positive and negative aspects of the mentorship relationship and argue that the relationship can be emotionally draining, especially when things go wrong, and like a lot of emotional work the effort and labour is often unacknowledged (Hochschild, 1983). They also go on to consider the student, and part of the mentorship relationship is that the student must engage and be seen to be bright and enthusiastic and to want to fit in with the practice setting; they must therefore engage with a degree of impression management (Goffman, 1959). Whilst this is inevitable and arguably even desirable, an important issue is that when dealing with the student who is perceived to be difficult or challenging the mentor does reflect on what the area of difficulty is; is it because the student does not fit in with the mentor's idea of how the student should dress or conduct themselves or is it because of a specific weakness?

The Nursing and Midwifery Council produced a report written by Kathleen Duffy (Duffy, 2004) entitled 'Failing Students'. It was based on her research study in which she examined the experience of the underperforming student in clinical practice, and although it was concerned with nursing students it has implications for all health professions. She identified a number of issues, one of which was that the mentor of the students will need support in handling and in dealing with this type of situation. Help can be sought from a variety of sources, such as experienced colleagues. Importantly, the university or educational establishment the student attends should provide support (Watson, 2000).

To reiterate, it is important to identify exactly what the issue or difficulty is, the more precisely the better, and a detailed individual action plan can be drawn up to begin to address these areas of difficulty. Duffy (2004) did identify the main areas of difficulty as being interpersonal skills and technical skills. As soon as it becomes apparent that there may be a problem, an action plan needs to be developed and there is a need for regular review and careful monitoring of the situation. Duffy makes the point that often people leave it too late before taking action – the sooner the student is advised of the perceived problem the better. Many people can be helped and assisted at this stage.

The whole aim of this aspect of the mentorship process is to help the individual. The first step is to talk to the student to find out what the difficulties are and their perceptions of the problem, and with them develop an action plan. Encourage students to look at their learning and learning strategies; work out with them some very concrete steps that they can take to address their particular difficulties and set targets and be clear about these targets so it is easy to determine that they have achieved these targets. This is where help and support is useful. Do get help; it might be someone to discuss strategies used or it may be someone coming to meetings with the student and the mentor. It is important that everything about progress to date is carefully documented. All of this will take time and it needs to be discussed with your manager and extra time might need to be negotiated to complete this.

Despite all these efforts not all students will demonstrate competency at the end of the placement and it is important that the student is not passed. There is much evidence that, in this situation, many people are passing rather than failing the student. It is, of course pleasanter and in many ways more rewarding to pass but only if justified. Mentors are professionals and bound by professional codes which they must follow. It is also important to recognise that these situations are stressful for the mentor and the importance of talking things through with senior colleagues cannot be over emphasised.

The student with specific learning needs

You may find students in the clinical area with specific learning difficulties and these have been identified as **dyslexia**, **dyspraxia** and **dyscalculia**. Universities have for a number of years been developing approaches and strategies to help people with specific learning needs and there are challenges in practice. The first point is that in any profession students must be fit for practice, a disability is no barrier to successful practice but reasonable adjustments and strategies may need to be made to overcome these particular issues. In the UK the Disability Discrimination Act (1995) states that reasonable adjustment should be taken to overcome difficulties. Many people will come with specific action plans which indicate ways in which difficulties can be overcome, but what is important is that the mentor works with the individual to devise and develop strategies. It is also important to recognise the positive aspects, that many people with particular disabilities are very empathetic as they have to overcome many obstacles; they also tend to see the needs of patients holistically.

Dyslexia, dyscalculia and dyspraxia

In this section the ways in which people with these particular difficulties can be assisted will be explored. There is also information available on the web which is very helpful; in particular, the Royal College of Nursing have produced a tool kit (Cowan, 2010) which gives an excellent overview and it also highlights a number of strategic approaches which can be taken to assist and support the learners.

The Dyslexia Institute has defined dyslexia as follows:

Dyslexia causes difficulties in learning to read, write and spell. Short-term memory, mathematics, concentration, personal organisation may also be affected. Dyslexia usually arises from a weakness in the processing of language-based information.

Biological in origin, it tends to run in families, but environmental factors also contribute. Dyslexia can occur at any level of intellectual ability. It is not the result of poor motivation, emotional disturbance, sensory impairment or lack of opportunities, but it may occur alongside any of these. The effects of dyslexia can be largely overcome by skilled specialist teaching and the use of compensatory strategies.

(Dyslexia Institute, 2000)

It is important to note that dyslexia does not only involve reading difficulties but can affect short-term memory and numeracy; it can also be mild, moderate and severe and often people with dyslexia are average or above average in intelligence. Dyslexia is no barrier to successful practice, and in reality people with dyslexia have had to develop coping strategies and means of overcoming their particular difficulties, and they often bring a range of skills to the clinical environment which can enhance patient safety (Davis & Baum, 1997). Whilst dyslexia is the commonest issue, two other often associated areas are dyscalculia and dyspraxia.

The Department for Education and Science (2001) defines dyscalculia as:

A condition that affects the ability to acquire arithmetical skills. Dyscalculic learners may have difficulty understanding simple number concepts, lack an intuitive grasp of numbers, and have problems learning number facts and procedures. Even if they produce a correct answer or use a correct method, they may do so mechanically and without confidence.

According to the British Dyslexia Association 40–50% of people with dyslexia will have dyscalculia as well; however very few people are found to have true dyscalculia, whereas many people are simply bad at mathematics and can improve. People with dyscalculia will have difficulties with numbers and will also have time related difficulties. What are particularly important are drug calculations. In their toolkit they suggested that people with dyspraxia will need specialist assistance but those with dyslexia or dyspraxia may find particular strategies helpful, such as checking answers with a calculator, carrying formulae around with them, continual practice and possibly attendance at adult numeracy classes (Cowan, 2010).

Dyspraxia has been defined as:

Developmental dyspraxia is an impairment or immaturity of the organisation of movement. It is an immaturity in the way that the brain processes information, which results in messages not being properly or fully transmitted. The term dyspraxia comes from the word praxis, which means 'doing, acting'. Dyspraxia affects the planning of what to do and how to do it. It is associated with problems of perception, language and thought...
(The Dyspraxia Foundation,
available at www. dyspraxiafoundation.org.uk, accessed 15/05/12.)

Cowan (2010) suggests that the particular difficulties people with dyspraxia will have are poor concentration, inappropriately loud speech, co-ordination difficulties, emotional and perceptual problems.

It is important that people working with the individual are made aware of their condition and this particularly applies to practice (Dale & Atkin, 2007). Practice areas should be made aware of the student's needs and in particular before the student arrives on placement; this necessitates disclosure to which the student must agree. There is no legal requirement that the student discloses their disability, although as they will receive specialist help it is clearly in their interest to do so.

It is the theme of this chapter that 'good mentorship is good mentorship' and this maxim very much applies to this situation. However, it is important that the mentor has knowledge about the student with particular difficulties and is happy to work with the student to explore strategies for overcoming any difficulties; this necessitates time and also outside help. The mentor should discuss any issues and concerns with the student's tutor. Whilst universities have well recognised and good support, in all probability this will not be replicated in the clinical setting: It is also only in the past ten years or so that many of these issues have been recognised and discussed. It should be noted however that students are not required to disclose disability, and this in itself can bring challenges.

There are various strategies people can use to overcome these difficulties and students may need a degree of specialist support and assistance and more opportunities to practice. If you are required to mentor a student with any of these conditions, the student often comes with an action plan which highlights the areas and has strategies in place to address specific needs.

White (2007) highlights some of the difficulties which can be experienced in clinical work; she is writing from a nursing perspective but many of these issues apply to other professional groups. It is also important to emphasise that not everyone who is dyslexic will experience problems. Difficulties can fall into the following main areas:

Language skills: the difficulties are around language skills, spelling, reading aloud, and writing in front of others.

Dealing with information: particularly at handovers where information may be conveyed quickly; completing records, for example, patient reports where there may be a degree of pressure to get the job done quickly and accurately. Unfamiliar terminology may also be difficult when first heard. Unfamiliar drug names may be problematic.

Role function: issues around dealing with instructions, remembering to do things, prioritising tasks – all may pose a challenge.

Tasks involving numeracy: such as administration of drugs – calculating drug doses.

Together the student and mentor can work out strategies to overcome particular problems and in addition to the support which can be offered by educational institutions there are a number of resources available, such as the RCN Toolkit (Cowan, 2010), and published material such as Illingworth (2005); in Table 6.1, Illingworth (2005) lists particular difficulties and strategies which people may take to overcome these difficulties. Other suggestions are available from Cowan (2010) and the associated literature.

Table 6.1 Strategies for overcoming obstacles *(Illingworth 2005)*

Obstacle	Strategy
Filling in forms	Become familiar with forms so know what to fill in; get forms checked; ask someone else to fill in form
Lose concentration when writing report	Leave it and come back later
Remembering people's names	Repeat many times after meeting them
Remembering verbal instructions	Always have paper in pocket for notes
Spelling	Be aware of problem words, ask someone how to spell them, use memory techniques, dictionary, spell checker.
Taking and organising messages	Ask caller to speak slowly, read back messages over phone to double check, and keep all messages and results in one place.
Taking notes in lectures, and meetings	Develop own shorthand, pick out key points, use dictaphone, use handouts when available.
Writing letters, e-mails, records and reports	Use set documentation, use set phrases, write things out in rough first, and get things checked before they are sent out, read novels to experience different types of writing.

Whilst people can experience difficulties in a variety of situations, it is worth highlighting medication administration. Firstly, true dyscalculia is relatively uncommon, and most people will come with a specific action plan to address any difficulties. People with dyslexia may experience difficulties with calculations and many are simply bad at maths. As there are a number of safety implications it is an area which must be taken very seriously. Cowan (2010: 33) has listed a number of strategies which may be helpful to colleagues. The following box provides a summary of these points.

- Allow individuals to work at their own pace.

- Provide clinical examples.

- Help colleagues to feel open about asking for help.

- Encourage students to look at books available on nursing calculations.

- Give concrete examples.

- Encourage use of calculators.

Conclusion

This chapter has considered students who may have particular needs and issues that must be addressed in order for them to work towards achieving their learning goals.

We are reminded by Biggs (1999) that good mentorship is good mentorship regardless of context and if the principles of mentorship are followed many difficult or taxing situations can be resolved easily.

Finally, remember that as a mentor you are not working in isolation and where you are experiencing difficulties it is best to discuss this with a senior colleague or the appropriate staff member in the university or college, sooner rather than later.

References

Allen, T.D., Finkelstein, L.M., & Poteet, M.L. (2009) *Designing Workplace Mentoring Programs: An Evidence-based Approach*. Oxford: Wiley-Blackwell.

Anderson, E., Manek, N. & Davidson, A. (2006) 'Evaluation of a model for maximizing interprofessional education in an acute hospital' in *Journal of Interprofessional Care*, **20**(2): 182–194.

Andrews, M., & Wallis, M. (1999). 'Mentorship in nursing: a literature review' in *Journal of Advanced Nursing*, **29**(1): 201–207.

Atkins, S. & Murphy, K. (1993) 'Reflection: A review of the literature' in *Journal of Advanced Nursing*, **18**: 118–119.

Bandura, A. (1994) 'Self-efficacy' in *Encyclopaedia of Human Behaviour*, ed. V.S. Ramachandran, **4**, 71–81. New York: Academic Press.

Barnett, N. (2011) 'Just started a new job? Or is work a bit tough?: You might profit from a mentor' in *Pharmaceutical Journal* **286** (7641): 202–203.

Baumard, P. (1999) *Tacit Knowledge in Organisations*. London: Sage.

Benner, P. (1984) *From Novice to Expert: Excellence and Power in Clinical Nursing Practice*. Jersey: Addison-Wesley.

Bhatti, N. & Viney, R. (2010) 'Coaching and mentoring' in *British Medical Journal*, **341**(7764): 21–23.

Biggs, J. (1999) *Teaching for Quality Learning at University*. Buckingham: Society for Research into Higher Education: Open University Press.

Biggs, J. (2003) *Teaching for Quality in Higher Education* Maidenhead; Open University Press

Boud, D. & Solomon, N. (eds) (2001) *Work-based Learning: A New Higher Education?* Buckingham: Open University Press.

Bray, L. & Nettleton, P. (2007) 'Assessor or mentor? Role confusion in professional education' in *Nurse Education Today*, **27**(8): 848–855.

Brennan, J. & Little, B. (2010) 'Graduate competences and relationships with the labour market: the UK case' in *Development of Competencies in the World of Work and Education*, paper presented at conference: Ljubljana, Slovenia.

Bulut, H., Hisar, F. & Demir, S.G. (2010) 'Evaluation of mentorship programme in nursing education: a pilot study in Turkey' in *Nurse Education Today* **30**(8): 756–762.

Burnard, P. (1989) *Know Yourself! Self Awareness Activities for Nurses*. London: Scutari Press.

Cammish, N.K. (1997) 'Through a glass darkly: problems of studying at advanced level through the medium of English' in *Overseas Students in Higher Education: Issues in Teaching and Learning*, eds. D. McNamara and R. Harris. London: Routledge, pp. 143–155.

Carlisle, C., Calman, L. & Ibbotson, T. (2009) 'Practice-based learning: The role of practice education facilitators in supporting mentors' in *Nurse Education Today* **29**: 715–721.

Chambers, B. (2010) 'Something to aspire to' in *Health Service Journal*, **120** (6215): 22.

Clark, P. (2006) 'What would a theory of inter-professional education look like? Some suggestions for developing a theoretical framework for teamwork training' in *Journal of Inter-professional Care*, **20**(6): 577–589.

Clutterbuck, D. & Megginson, D. (2009) *Further Techniques for Coaching and Mentoring*. London: Butterworth-Heinemann.

Cortazzi, M. & Jin, L. (1997) 'Communication for learning across cultures' in D. McNamara & R. Harris (eds.), *Overseas Students in Higher Education* (pp. 76–90). London and New York: Routledge.

Cowan, M. (2010) *Dyslexia, Dyscalculia and Dyspraxia. A Toolkit for Nursing Staff*. London: Royal College of Nursing.

Cornford, I. R., (2000) Learning-to-learn Skills for Lifelong Learning: Some Implications for Curriculum Development and Teacher Education. Available at www.aare.edu.au/00pap/cor00382.htm (accessed 15/07/12.)

Dale, C. & Aiken, F. (2007) *A Review of the Literature into Dyslexia in Nursing Practice*. London: RCN.

Daroszewski, E. B. (2004) 'Commentary by Daroszewski' in *Western Journal of Nursing Research*, **26**: 170–172.

Davis, R.D. & Baum, E.M. (1997) *The Gift of Dyslexia: Why some of the Smartest People Can't Read and How They Can Learn*. London: Souvenir Press.

Department for Education and Science (2001) Available at: www.reading.ac.uk/disability/about/DyslexiaSLDs/do-dyscalculia.aspx (accessed 17/07/12).

Dewey, D. (1933) *How We Think*. Boston: DC Health.

Dewing, J. (1990) 'After primary nursing- what next?' in *Nursing* **4**(25): 16–18.

Disability Discrimination Act (1995) Available at: www.legislation.gov.uk/pga/1995/50/contents (accessed 17/07/12).

Downie, C.M. & Basford, P. (1998) *Teaching and Assessing in Clinical Practice. A Reader.* 2nd edn. London: The University of Greenwich.

Duffy, K. (2004) *Failing Students: A Qualitative Study of Factors that Influence the Decisions Regarding Assessment of Students' Competence in Practice*. London: NMC.

Durrant, A., Rhodes, G. & Young, D. (eds) (2009) *Getting Started with University-Level Work Based Learning*. London: Middlesex University Press.

Dyslexia Institute (2002) Available at: http://www.beingdyslexic.co.uk/pages/information/general-information/dyslexia-basics/what-is-dyslexia.php (accessed 15/07/12).

Dyspraxia Foundation (n.d.) Available at: http://www.dyspraxiafoundation.org.uk/services/dys_dyspraxia.php (accessed 15/07/12).

Equality Act (2010) Available at: http://www.homeoffice.gov.uk/equalities/equality-strategy/ (accessed 17/07/12).

Flanaghan, J. (1954) 'The critical incident technique' in *Psychological Bulletin* **51**(4): 327–358.

Fulton, J., Buhler, A., Hansen, G.S., Kauffeldt, A., Welander, E., Santos, M.R., Thorarinsdottir, K. & Ziarko, E. (2007) 'Mentorship: An international perspective' in *Nurse Education in Practice* **7**(6): 399–406.

Furnham, A. & Bochner, S. (1986) *Culture Shock: Psychological Reactions to Unfamliar Environments*. London: Methuen & Co. Ltd.

Galtung, J. (1981) 'Structure, culture, and intellectual style: An essay comparing saxonic, teutonic, gallic and nipponic approaches' in *Social Science Information*, **20**(6): 817–856.

Gay, G. (2000) *Culturally Responsive Teaching: Theory, Research and Practice*. Columbia University New York: Teacher College Press.

Ghaye, T. & Lillyman, S. (2000) *Reflection: Principles and Practice for Healthcare Professionals*. Dinton: Quay Books/Mark Allen.

Gibbs., G. (1988) *Learning by Doing*. Oxford: Further Education Unit, Oxford Polytechnic.

Goffman, E. (1959) *The Presentation of Self in Everyday Life*. New York: Anchor Books.

Goodman., J. (1984) 'Reflection and teacher education: a case study and reciprocal analysis' in *Interchange* **15**(3): 9–26.

Gosling, D. & Moon, J. (2002) *Learning How to Use Learning Outcomes and Assessment Criteria*, 3rd edn. London: SEEC.

Gustafsson, C. & Fagerberg, I. (2004) 'Reflection, the way to professional development?' in *Journal of Clinical Nursing*, **13**(3): 271–280.

Higher Education Academy (HEA) (2007) Workshop material presented at University of Sunderland, 2007.

Hochschild, A.R. (1983) *The Managed Heart: Commercialisation of Human Feeling.* Berkeley, CA: University of California Press.

Honey, P. & Mumford, A. (1989) 'Setting the scene for learning' in Downie, C.M. & Basford, P, (2003) *Mentoring in Practice. A Reader*. London: The University of Greenwich.

Howatson-Jones, L. (2010) *Reflective Practice in Nursing (Transforming Nursing Practice)*. Exeter: Learning Matters.

Hyland, T. (1994) *Competence, Education and NVQs. Dissenting Perspectives*. London: Cassell Education.

Ibarra, H. (1999) 'Provisional selves: experimenting with image and identity in professional adaptation' in *Administrative Science Quarterly*, **44**(4): 764–791.

Illingworth, K. (2005) 'The effects of dyslexia on the work of nurses and healthcare assistants' in *Nursing Standard*, **19**(38): 41–48.

Insch, G.S., McIntyre, N. & Dawley, D. (2008) 'Tacit knowledge: A refinement and empirical test of the academic tacit knowledge scale' in *Journal of Psychology* **142**(6): 561–579.

Irons, A. (2008) *Enhancing Learning Through Formative Assessment and Feedback*. London: Routledge.

Jasper, M. (2003) *Beginning Reflective Practice – Foundations in Nursing and Healthcare*. Cheltenham: Nelson Thorne.

Jefferies, A. & Skidmore, M. (2010)'Evaluation of a collaborative mentorship program in a multi-site postgraduate training program' in *Medical Teacher*, **32**(8): 695–697.

Jokelainen, M., Turunen, H., Tossavainen, K., Jamookeeah, D. & Coco, K. (2011) 'A systematic review of mentoring nursing students in clinical placements' in *Journal of Clinical Nursing* 1-14 (published online).

Jones, S., Maxfield, M. & Levington, A. (2010) 'A mentor portfolio model for ensuring fitness for practice' in *Nursing Management*, **16** (10): 28–31.

Kadivar, H. (2010) 'The importance of mentorship for success in family medicine' in *Annals of Family Medicine* **8**(4): 374–375.

Knowles, M. (1984) *The Adult Learner: A Neglected Species*, 3rd edn. Houston: Gulf Publishing Company.

Kolb, D. (1984) *Experiential Learning: Experience as the Source of Learning and Development*. Englewood Cliffs NJ: Prentice Hall.

Kostovich, C. (2010). 'Becoming a nurse researcher: the importance of mentorship' in *Nursing Science Quarterly*, **23**(4): 281–286.

Lave, J. & Wenger, E. (1991) *Situated Learning: Legitimate Peripheral Participation*. Cambridge: Cambridge University Press.

Lewin, D. (2007) 'Clinical learning environments for student nurses: key indices from two studies compared over a 25 year period' in *Nurse Education in Practice* **7**(4): 238–246.

Li, Y.S., Chen, H.M., Yang, B.H. & Liu, C.F. (2011) 'An exploratory study of the relationships between age and learning styles among students in different nursing programmes in Taiwan' in *Nurse Education Today*, **31**(1): 18–23.

Luzio-Lockett, A. (1998) 'The squeezing effect: the cross-cultural experience of international students' in *British Journal of Guidance & Counselling* **26**(2): 209–223.

Macafee, D. & Garvey, B. (2010) 'Mentoring and coaching: What's the difference?' in *British Medical Journal*, **341**(7764): 22–23.

McKenna, G. (1995) 'Learning Theories Made Easy: Cognitivism' in *Mentoring in Practice. A Reader* (2003), eds C.M. Downie & P. Basford. London: The University of Greenwich, p. 101.

McNett, J.M., Wallace, R.M. & Athanassiou, N. (2004) 'Tacit knowledge in the classroom: A strategy for learning', Paper presented at 29th Improving University Teaching conference, Bern, Switzerland.

Marshall, M. & Gordon, F. (2010) 'Exploring the role of the inter-professional mentor' in *Journal of Inter-professional Care*, **24**(4): 362–374.

Marton,, F. & Salvo, J. (1976a) 'On qualitative differences in learning I, outcome and process' in *British Journal of Educational Psychology* **46**: 4–11.

Marton, F., Salvo, J. (1976b) 'On qualitative differences in learning II, outcome as a function of learners' perception of the task' in *British Journal of Educational Psychology* **46**: 4–11.

Maslow, A. H. (1971) *The Farther Reaches of Human Nature*. New York: Esalen Books, Viking Press.

Mead, G. H. (1934) *Mind, Self and Society: From the Standpoint of a Social Behaviourist*. University of Chicago Press: Chicago.

Meehan-Andrews, T.A. (2008) 'Teaching mode efficiency and learning preferences of first year nursing students' in *Nurse Education Today*, **29**(1): 24–32.

Merriam, S. & Caffarella, S. (1991) *Learning in Adulthood. A Comprehensive Guide*. San Francisco: Jossey-Bass.

Mezirow, J. (1981) 'A critical theory of adult learning and education' in *Adult Education Quarterly*, **32**(1): 3–24.

Mitchell, J. T. & Everly, G. S. (1993) *Critical Incident Stress Debriefing (CISD): An operations manual for the prevention of traumatic stress among emergency services and disaster workers*. USA. Chevron.

Moon, J. (2006) *A Handbook of Reflective and Experiential Learning: Theory and Practice*. London: Routledge Falmer.

Nash, S. & Scammell, J. (2010) 'Skills to ensure success in mentoring and other workplace learning approaches' in *Nursing Times*, **106** (2): 17–20.

Nasir, S.N. & Hand, V. (2006) 'Exploring sociocultural perspectives on race, culture and learning' in *Review of Educational Research*, **76**(4): 449–475.

Nonaka, I. (2007) 'The knowledge creating company' in *Harvard Business Review* Jul-Aug.

Nursing and Midwifery Council (NMC) (2008) *Standards to Support Learning and Assessment in Practice. NMC standards for mentors, practice teachers and teachers*. London: NMC.

Nursing and Midwifery Council (NMC) (2010) *Standards for Pre-registration Nursing Education*. London: NMC.

Overton, G.K., Kelly, D., McCallister, P., Jones, J. & MacVicar, R. (2009) 'The practice-based small group learning approach: making evidence-based practice come alive for learners' in *Nurse Education Today*, **29**(6): 671–675.

Paget, T. (2001) 'Reflective practice and clinical outcomes: practitioners' views on how reflective practice has influenced their clinical practice' in *Journal of Clinical Nursing*, **10**(2): 204–214.

Pearcey, P.A., Elliott, B.E. (2004) 'Student impressions of clinical nursing' in *Nurse Education Today*, **24**(5): 382–387.

Polanyi, M. (1998) *Personal Knowledge: Towards a Post Critical Philosophy*. London: Routledge.

Quality Assurance Agency for Higher Education (QAA) (2008) *The Framework for Higher Education Qualifications in England, Wales and Northern Ireland*. Mansfield: The Quality Assurance Agency for Higher Education.

Rogers, C. (1983) *Freedom to learn for the 80's*. Columbus, Ohio: Merrill Publishing Company.

Rotter, J. (1966), 'Generalized expectancies of internal versus external control of reinforcements' in *Psychological Monographs, The American Psychological Association* **80**(1), 1966; 1–28.

Sadler, R. (2009) 'Fidelity as a precondition for integrity in grading academic achievement' in *Assessment and Evaluation in Higher Education*, **35**: 727–743.

Sanders, G. (2010) 'Towards a model of multi-organisational work-based learning: developmental networks as a mechanism for tacit knowledge transfer and exploration of professional identity' in *Learning and Teaching in Higher Education* **4**(1).

Scanlan, J.M., Care, W.D. & Udod, S. (2002) 'Unravelling the unknowns of reflection in classroom teaching' in *Journal of Advanced Nursing*, **38**(4): 136–143.

Scardamalia, M., Bereiter, C., Brett, C., Burtis, P.J., Calhoun, C. & Smith Lea, N. (1992) 'Educational applications of a networked communal database' in *Interactive Learning Environments*, **2**(1): 45–71.

Schon, D. A. (1983) *The Reflective Practitioner: How Professionals Think in Action*. London: Temple Smith.

Schon, D. (1987) *Educating the Reflective Practitioner*. San Francisco: Jossey-Bass.

Shakespeare, P. & Webb, C. (2008) 'Professional identity as a resource for talk: Exploring the mentor-student relationship' in *Nursing Inquiry* **15**(4): 270–279).

Sternberg, R.J. & Wagner, R.K. (1993) 'The g-ocentric view of intelligence and job performance is wrong' in *Current Directions in Psychological Science* **2**(1): 1–5.

Sternberg, R.J. & Horvath, J.A. (1999) *Tacit Knowledge in Professional Practice: Researcher and Practitioner Perspectives*. Mahwah, NJ: Lawrence Erlbaum Associates.

Taylor, P.G. (1999) *Making Sense of Academic Life: Academics, Universities and Change*. Buckingham: Open University Press.

Thomas-Maclean, R., Hamoline, R., Quinlan, E., Ramsden, V.R. & Kuzmicz, J. (2010) 'Discussing mentorship: an ongoing study for the development of a mentorship program in Saskatchewan', *Canadian Family Physician*, Nov; **19**(11): 1205–12.

Torrance, H. & Pryor, J. (2002) *Investigating Formative Assessment, Teaching and Learning in the Classroom*. Buckingham: Open University Press, McGraw Hill.

Vaughn, L.M., Battle, J.M., Taylor, T. & Dearman, L. (2009) 'Learning styles and the relationship to attachment styles and psychological symptoms in college women' in *College Student Journal*, **43**(3): 723–735.

Vygotsky, L.S. (1978) *Mind and Society: The Development of Higher Psychological Processes*. Cambridge, MA: Harvard University Press.

Wagner, R.K. (1987) 'Tacit knowledge in everyday intelligent behaviour' in *Journal of Personality and Social Psychology*, **52** (6): 1236–1247.

Watson, S. (2000) 'The support that mentors receive in the clinical setting' in *Nurse Education Today*, **20**(7): 585–592.

Wenger, E. (2008) *Communities of Practice. Learning, Meaning and Identity*. New York: Cambridge University Press.

White, J. (2007) 'Supporting nursing students with dyslexia in clinical practice' in *Nursing Standard*, **21**(19): 35–42.

Wilkinson, C., Peters, L., Mitchell, K., Irwin, T., McCorrie, K. & MacLeod, M. (1998) ' "Being there": learning through active participation' in *Nurse Education Today*, **18**(3): 223–230.

Yang, C.L., Wei, S.T. (2010) 'Modelling the performance of CoP in knowledge management' in *Total Quality Management and Business Excellence*, **21**(9): 1033–1045.

Index